WRITING USEFUL, ACCESSIBLE, AND LEGALLY DEFENSIBLE

PSYCHOEDUCATIONAL REPORTS

MICHAEL R. HASS
JEANNE ANNE M. CARRIERE

WILEY

Library of Congress Cataloging-in-Publication Data:

Hass, Michael R.
    Writing useful, accessible, and legally defensible psychoeducational reports / Michael R. Hass, Ph.D.,
Jeanne Anne M. Carriere, Ph.D. — 1
        pages cm
    Includes bibliographical references and index.
    ISBN 978-1-118-20565-5 (pbk.); ISBN 978-1-118-82494-8 (ebk); ISBN 978-1-118-85239-2 (ebk)
        1. Individualized education programs.   2. Report writing.   3. Children with disabilities —
Education — Evaluation.   I. Carriere, Jeanne Anne M.   II. Title.
    LC4019.H384 2014
    371.2 — dc23

                                                                                    2013044598

Printed in the United States of America

SKY10067149_021224

For our students: Your intelligence, commitment,
and tolerance for ambiguity continually inspire us to be the
best practitioners and professors we can be.
—MH & JAC

For my trinity of mentors: Steven Hodge for lighting the fire, Judy McBride
for providing the fuel, and Michael Hass for modeling containment and escalation
methods for a long and memorable burn.
—JAC

Contents

Acknowledgments

We feel a great deal of gratitude for the family, friends, and colleagues who have supported us through this process. Thank you to our editor, Marquita Flemming, who initially proposed this book. Her vision, patience, and guidance have been our driving force.

A big thank-you to Patricia Harriman and our Wiley "editing crew." We are also indebted to our colleagues, Kelly Kennedy and John Brady, who provided lightning-fast comments and critique. This is a better book because of all their efforts.

A special thank-you to all of our colleagues in the Counseling and School Psychology Program, whose collegiality, support, and wicked sense of humor keep us from taking ourselves too seriously.

Michael would like to thank Gabrielle for her faith in his abilities and for always meeting the statement "I have to work on the book" with encouragement and support.

Jeanne Anne thanks her husband, Steve, and daughters, Lila and Scarlett, for their understanding of her recent long hours and their loving encouragement when deadlines loomed. She would also like to thank her parents, who have always been her biggest supporters.

Finally, we thank our readers. We sincerely hope you will find this book useful.

WRITING USEFUL, ACCESSIBLE, AND LEGALLY DEFENSIBLE

PSYCHOEDUCATIONAL REPORTS

Why Is Another Book on Report Writing Needed?

Jeanne Anne's husband is a teacher. Early in their relationship, as she was spending her Saturday afternoon writing psychoeducational reports, he flippantly asked, "Why are you spending so much time on those? Nobody reads them anyway." At the time, her frustration hindered her ability to engage in a meaningful conversation about his opinion, probably because at some level she knew he was correct. She truly had become a gatekeeper on the way to Special Education services and her report was simply a step to be completed. It had no purpose other than to sit in a file. A seed was planted, and what would become a professional journey to improve the usefulness of her reports began. Along the way she met Michael, whose journey probably began on a much less dramatic note. He was spending a lot of time and effort on his assessments, had important to things to say, and wanted people to read his reports and consider his recommendations.

This book is the result of our efforts both as practitioners to write better reports and as educators to teach others to do so as well. Our goal for our students and ourselves is to write reports that represent children and their needs in a way that is useful to the stakeholders involved with those children, especially parents and teachers. Recognizing that special education has become increasingly litigious, we also want those reports to reflect the ethical and legal demands and constraints put upon us by our professional standards as well as state and federal laws and regulations. Our position is that we can accomplish both and it is not necessary to sacrifice usefulness and accessibility to meet legal and ethical mandates. We take this a step further and argue that making our reports more accessible and useful to consumers will itself make them more ethical and legally compliant.

We have written and read many psychological reports during careers that between us span over 40 years of experience as practitioners and 26 years as trainers of school psychologists. During that time, we estimate that we have written over a thousand psychological reports and read at least that many of our students' reports. As university trainers, we have also read reports from dozens of local school districts. Things have changed considerably over our careers. When Jeanne Anne began her first school psychology job in 1993, she created hand-written reports using a three-page template, essentially a psychological fill-in-the-blank format. When Michael began his career, several years before Jeanne Anne, his reports were also handwritten, but the fill-in-the-blank template was only two pages long. It is clear to us that these early efforts at representing children in a written document contained very little information that was useful to parents or educators. Currently, we work in an area of the country where 30- to 50-page reports based on highly detailed templates is the norm. Unfortunately, we often find these much longer documents still do not contain much that is truly useful to parents and teachers.

A few years ago, we took the ideas we had developed as practitioners and trainers and created a workshop that we then presented at local, state, and national conferences. To our surprise, these workshops were often filled to capacity, frequently with people sitting on the floor around the edges of the room. This taught us that although practitioners write many reports, they are not necessarily confident in their skills. We also discovered that practitioners write reports with a striking range of formats and lengths.

We have noted a trend toward writing longer, less comprehensible reports in the name of legal defensiveness. We believe that most of these reports have several problems that hinder their usefulness to readers and actually make them less legally defensible. For example, they often lack focus and cohesiveness, have little actual interpretation, do not provide useful recommendations, and use vocabulary that only professionals with graduate degrees could possibly understand. They are also typically full of boilerplate legal language that does not appear to serve any useful purpose, including that of making the assessment or report more legally defensible. In addition to this legal filler language, a concerned parent or teacher often has to wade through many vague and generic statements that could be about nearly any child assessed to discover useful information unique to the specific child they are concerned about.

One goal in writing this book is to push back against this trend. We challenge the notion that longer is better and that the way we conduct our assessments and write reports should be guided by fear of legal action. Simply put, we believe that an assessment that directly responds to the concerns of parents and teachers and a report that communicates the results of that assessment in a way that the reader can easily understand is not only best practice but also easier to legally defend than the 40- or 50-page monster reports we often see. This book represents our current best thinking about how to accomplish this. As we explain in detail later in the book, the model we propose is based on a synthesis of published research, an analysis of professional guidelines, reflections on our own experience writing reports and teaching report writing, and what one of our colleagues calls *PJs* (professional judgments).

In this book, we advocate for question-driven assessments and suggest that these questions serve to frame reports. In that spirit, we have structured the book in the same way. Each chapter begins with a question. For example, the title of this chapter is "Why is another book on report writing needed?" Following that, we have a series of sections and subsections that we conceptualize as follow-up questions and themes. *Theme statements* are concise statements that summarize the major finding of the information that follows. This also follows the structure we advocate for reports. In Chapter 1, the themes include: (a) Report writing is important; (b) Assessment and report writing consumes a lot of our time and is a fundamental task of school psychologists; and (c) Reports should clearly communicate important information to consumers that makes a difference in the lives of the children involved.

We have used many examples to illustrate our points throughout this book, including six sample reports in Appendix II. To preserve the confidentiality of those involved, we have changed all identifying information and used pseudonyms for the personal names, schools, school districts, and agencies discussed. To retain a level of authenticity, some examples contain actual assessment instruments. By including them in our examples, we are not endorsing or opposing the use of these instruments.

REPORT WRITING IS IMPORTANT

Throughout this book, we will discuss assessment as well as report writing. The reason for this is that the two cannot be separated. As succinctly stated by Brown-Chidsey and Steege, "No assessment is likely to be useful until, or unless, the findings are communicated to those in a position to implement solutions" (2005, p. 267). The value of a well-designed and focused assessment is easily obscured by a poorly organized and written report and, conversely, a poorly designed assessment cannot be rescued by a beautifully written report. School psychology graduate programs pay considerable attention to assessment but, if judged by the practitioners who attend our workshops, less attention to report writing.

Assessment can be defined as the process of gathering information to inform decisions (Salvia, Ysseldyke, & Bolt, 2007). No matter your philosophy about what constitutes a valid or useful assessment, the process involves collecting and evaluating data for the purpose of responding to stakeholders' questions and concerns, identifying needs and strengths, and making meaningful recommendations. These data are also used to make decisions regarding further assessment, diagnosis or disability classification, and instructional planning (Salvia, Ysseldyke, & Bolt, 2007; Sattler, 1992).

We argue that report writing is a critical yet undervalued part of the evaluation process. Unfortunately, practitioners often view report writing as a perfunctory post-assessment task. The report is sometimes completed the night before or even minutes before a meeting, without giving team members, including parents, the opportunity to review the findings before making critical decisions about the student's education. Although they are frequently not given the same attention as other aspects of the assessment process, psychological reports are important because they become the basis for the multidisciplinary teams' decisions regarding eligibility for special education and the foundation for recommending services and intervention. In other words, reports guide all of the decisions and planning that follow an assessment.

ASSESSMENT AND REPORT WRITING CONSUMES A LOT OF OUR TIME AND IS A FUNDAMENTAL TASK FOR SCHOOL PSYCHOLOGISTS

School psychology is a relatively young profession. Fagan and Wise (2000) conceptually divided the developmental history of school psychology into two eras. The first era, approximately the end of the 19th century to midway through the 20th century, was marked by widespread school reform. Early-20th-century political and sociocultural influences, specifically compulsory education laws, the corresponding increase in public school enrollment, and the development of intelligence testing, opened the door for the quantification of learning and achievement. This set the stage for the standardization of children's progress in school (Cook, 1912; Frey, 2005; National Conference of State Legislators, 2007). During this period, many types of educational and psychological practitioners provided services within the school setting. These services typically focused on assessment and diagnosis of learning difficulties.

The second era, midcentury to present, has seen the development of school psychologists' professional identity and an expansion of specialized training programs. For the first time, the majority of professionals practicing as school psychologists were trained in programs specifically designed for school psychologists. Throughout both of these eras, psychological assessment, diagnosis, and specialized program placement were the dominant roles of school psychologists (Fagan, 1990).

The results of several surveys of practitioners done over the last 40 years reflect this conclusion. In 1970, Farling and Hoedt (1971) conducted the first nationwide survey of school psychologists with the goal of identifying issues, concerns, and trends in the field. Their findings suggest that at that time the roles and functions of school psychologists were largely defined by assessment-related activities such as student evaluations, report writing, and parent–teacher meetings.

With the 1975 passage of the Education for All Handicapped Children Act (i.e., Public Law 94-142), it became public policy to educate children with disabilities at the public's expense.

PL 94-142 guaranteed parents of students with disabilities the right to be actively involved in their child's educational planning. They had the right to request assessment and, for the first time, had access to their children's records, including psychological reports (Weddig, 1984). Opinions regarding the impact this would have on the practice of school psychology were at opposite ends of the spectrum. Some thought the legislation would lead to more time spent on testing and other assessment activities while others predicted that it would lead to more opportunities for an expanded model of practice (Goldwasser, Meyers, Christenson, & Graden, 1983).

Eight years after the passing of PL 94-142, Goldwasser, Meyers, Christenson, and Graden (1983) undertook a national survey investigating school psychologists' perceptions of the legislation's impact on their roles. Respondents answered questions regarding evaluation procedures, Individualized Education Program (IEP) team membership, changes in role and function, due process participation, future training needs, and overall effects of the legislation. Two factors had negative implications for the psychologists' ability to engage in a broader range of services: an increased focus on students with disabilities, leading to limited opportunities to engage in preventative measures; and an increase in paperwork and administrative tasks, also reducing the time to engage in a wider range of professional activities. Surprisingly, the researchers found that the legislation had minimal impact on the overall roles of the respondents. School psychologists still spent the majority of their time engaged in diagnostic evaluations and related activities.

Researchers found similar survey results over the next 20 years. Smith (1984) surveyed a nationwide, random sample of school psychologists practicing in public school settings. Results indicated the majority of the psychologists' time was spent in assessment (54%), followed by intervention (23%), and consultation (19%). According to the survey results, school psychologists desired a reduction in assessment-based activities and an increase in intervention and consultation. In their survey of school psychology practitioners, Hutton, Dubes, and Muir (1992) reported that 53% of school psychologists' time was spent on assessment-related activities.

Clearly, research on the roles and functions of school psychologists suggests that assessment and related activities, including report writing, has shaped our practice throughout our century-long history (Curtis, Hunley, & Grier, 2002; Farling & Hoedt, 1971; Gilman & Medway, 2007; Hutton, Dubes, & Muir, 1992; Smith, 1984). Although school psychologists have a broad range of skills, we continue to be engaged in assessment-related endeavors more than in all other direct and indirect services combined. Given this, we know that for the vast majority of school psychologists, daily practice is still closely connected with assessment, diagnosis, and classification of students (Merrell, Ervin, & Gimpel, 2006). Indeed, in their comprehensive discussion of school psychology, Fagan and Wise (2000) contend that school psychologists' expertise in assessment has been the foundation of advancement and success in our field.

Over the last half century, many practitioners and researchers have called for an expansion of the role of school psychologists (Goldwasser, Meyers, Christenson, & Graden, 1983; Reschley, 2000). Shinn (2002) reported that school psychologists want to broaden their roles by increasing the time spent in non-assessment-related activities such as implementing social-emotional interventions, academic progress monitoring, and direct assessment methods. In 2006, Harvey surveyed 500 randomly selected members of the National Association of School Psychologists (NASP). Overall, the respondents indicated a desire to increase time spent outside of their traditional assessment role. Fifty-four percent of respondents wanted to increase their time spent in intervention progress monitoring, 48% wanted an increase in time spent on social and emotional interventions, and 56% wanted to increase their time spent in nontraditional assessment.

Given the longstanding and pervasive influence of assessment on the practice of school psychologists, the question is: Can this expertise be leveraged for more active involvement in prevention and intervention? NASP conceptualizes assessment as data-based decision making, and in the *Blueprint for Training and Practice III*, NASP defines competency in data-based decision making as the ability to accurately identify problems by gathering relevant data, then utilizing this integrated information in collaboration with others for better outcomes for students. NASP advocates for assessment to be conceptualized as a step in a problem-solving process that connects directly to prevention and intervention rather than a standalone activity (NASP, 2006).

We argue that psychological reports should reflect the dynamic nature of the problem-solving process and serve as a foundation for engaging in more consultation, prevention, and intervention. Bagnato (1980) has argued that psychological reports are the predominant way school psychologists demonstrate their value and effectiveness. The psychological report is a direct reflection of the quality and range of services school psychologists provide, and as the culminating activity of the problem-solving process, a well-conceptualized and well-written psychological report can be an important tool to expand our role and make our services more useful to parents and other educators.

REPORTS SHOULD CLEARLY COMMUNICATE INFORMATION TO CONSUMERS THAT MAKES A DIFFERENCE IN THE LIVES OF THE CHILDREN INVOLVED

In order to use reports as a tool to make ourselves more useful to parents and teachers, we must first understand what their purpose is. Ownby (1997) asserts that the purpose of a report is "to communicate assessment information in a fashion appropriate to the intended reader so that the reader's work with the client is affected" (p. 29). Although many individuals, including school administrators, outside professionals, and perhaps legal counsel, may read an assessment report hoping to better understand a child's strengths and needs, there is a strong argument that the most important consumers of psychological reports are the students' parents and teachers (Hagborg & Aiello-Coultier, 1994; Harvey, 1997; Weddig, 1984). Parents and teachers are the "front line" in the life of a child and the people most likely to both need and benefit from the information derived from an assessment.

It makes intuitive sense that a primary goal of psychological reports is to provide information that helps the people who live and work with children better understand their needs. Stated a different way, the goal of reports is to explicitly answer questions posed by those who referred the child for an assessment and to provide concrete recommendations (Eberst & Genshaft, 1984; Teglasi 1983). Although NASP has been relatively silent in regard to professional standards for report writing, in their *Principles for Professional Ethics and Guidelines for the Provision of School Psychological Services* (2010) they propose that assessment findings should be presented in language clearly understood by the recipient and that written reports should support the recipients in their work or interactions with the child. As school psychologists, we are expected not only to conduct assessments that address specific referral questions and interpret our findings in a meaningful way, but also to communicate that meaning in writing in a manner that others can understand.

If our objectives are to assist with educational planning and positively influence consumers' interactions with the student, we need to answer the question: How can we make the information in written psychological reports more useful and accessible to teachers and parents? Yet, the information needed to answer this question is sparse and not easily accessible (Ownby, 1997). For example, NASP has published a Best Practices in School Psychology series since 1985 (Thomas & Grimes, 1985), described as "a core resource on contemporary, evidence-based knowledge necessary for competent delivery of school psychological services" (NASP, 2009, para. 3). The first and second Best Practices editions had chapters dedicated to report writing but a chapter on report writing has not been included since the 1990 edition. This is despite the fact that with each new edition, the Best Practices volumes have grown exponentially, reaching 2,600 pages in the most recent fifth edition (Thomas & Grimes, 2008). These exclusions support our conviction that best practices are not clearly defined for report writing, a fundamental part of school psychologists' practice.

Although the assumption that school psychologists should write understandable and useful psychological reports is reflected in the NASP *Principles for Professional Ethics and Guidelines for the Provision of School Psychological Services* (2010), there is little specific guidance on how to accomplish this. For example, NASP guidelines state that assessment findings should be presented in language clearly understood by the recipients and that written reports should emphasize interpretation and recommendations to support the recipients in their work or interactions with the child. NASP clearly states that reports solely focusing on test scores or global statements are rarely useful yet provides little information on what the alternatives to these statements might be. We believe that this lack of clear consensus on the part of our profession is one reason that there is so much variability in reports and perhaps why supervisors of school psychologists have turned to attorneys and other people outside the profession to seek guidance on the best way to structure and write reports.

In the following chapters, we hope to fill this gap. In doing so, we also hope that our readers will take ownership of this important professional skill and learn not only to communicate clearly but to use their reports as a way to leverage a wider and more effective professional role.

We believe that report writing needs to be conceptualized as a vital part of the assessment process. We promote the use of question-driven assessments and reports as not only legally defensible, but also more accessible and useful for their most important consumers: educators and parents. As previously mentioned, the book follows the structure of a question-driven report. Each chapter title is a question and the headings within each chapter are strategic thematic statements that summarize key points. In Chapter 1, we answered the question, Why is another book on report writing needed? In the remaining chapters we address the following four questions: Chapter 2, What makes a report legally defensible?; Chapter 3, How do I make my reports more useful to consumers?; Chapter 4, Step-by-step, how do I write useful and legally defensible reports?; and Chapter 5, How do I solve practical problems along the way to question-driven report writing? At the end of the book, appendixes are included that provide tools to support a transition to more useful and legally defensible report writing, including a checklist to tell if your report is useful and legally defensible, extensive examples, and an interview protocol.

Chapter 1 Takeaway Points

- Although school psychologists have a broad range of skills, we continue to be engaged in assessment-related endeavors more than all other direct and indirect services combined.
- Psychoeducational reports are important because they become the basis for multidisciplinary teams' decisions regarding eligibility for special education and the foundation for recommending services and intervention.
- Report writing is a critical yet undervalued part of the evaluation process, often viewed as a perfunctory post-assessment task.

- The value of a well-designed and focused assessment can be easily obscured by a poorly organized and written report and, conversely, a poorly designed assessment cannot be rescued by a beautifully written report.
- We advocate for question-driven assessments and suggest that these questions serve to frame reports.
- The psychological report is a direct reflection of the quality and range of services school psychologists provide, and as the culminating activity of the problem-solving process, a well-conceptualized and well-written psychological report can be an important tool to expand our role and make our services more useful to parents and other educators.

What Makes a Report Legally Defensible?

Special education law is, if anything, complicated. Federal law contains many undefined terms and, in several places, appears to contradict itself (McBride, Dumont, & Willis, 2011). When you add the complexity of state regulations on top of this, it is no wonder that special education administrators often turn to attorneys for guidance in how to write legally defensible reports. Also making the task of sorting through federal special education law difficult is that there are several sources of legal guidance, including the Individuals with Disability Education Improvement Act of 2004 and the subsequent Final Regulations of 2006. Other sources include case law arising from circuit courts and Supreme Court decisions as well as various memos and letters from the Office of Special Education and Rehabilitative Services, the Office of Special Education Programs, and the Office of Civil Rights (McBride, Dumont, & Willis, 2011). In this chapter, we hope to provide clear characteristics of a legally defensible assessment and report by incorporating legal mandates with what we consider best practices.

The Education for All Handicapped Children Act (i.e., PL94-142) was amended, reauthorized, and renamed in 1997 and again in 2004. Now called the Individuals with Disabilities Education Act (IDEA), IDEA 2004 and the subsequent regulations provide the framework for parental involvement in children's educational decision making and planning. The law also secures parents' right to request an assessment and to be included in the IEP meeting to determine appropriate educational services for their child (IDEA 300.305; 300.306).

Interestingly, the federal laws and regulations have relatively little to say about reports. The evaluating agency is required to provide a copy of the evaluation report to the parent, but federal regulations do not determine a timeline for this. Given parents' right to inspect all relevant evaluations before a meeting, good practice and the spirit of the law suggest that they should be given copies of all reports before a meeting so they have the time to read and thoughtfully consider this information. This promotes parents' active participation in making decisions about their children's eligibility for special education services and developing the content of the IEP. Of course, even having sufficient time to read reports will have little benefit for parents if the reports are incomprehensible to them.

State laws and regulations can differ from federal law in that they sometimes have specific requirements for reports. For this reason, it is important to understand the legal mandates in the state(s) where you practice. For example, many Californians in our workshops are surprised to discover that the California Education Code (CEC) has several requirements for reports. These are examples of things that need to be addressed *explicitly* in reports. For example, CEC says that reports should include the following information (California Education Code Section 56327, a–g, 2009):

a. Does the student need special education and related services?
b. How was that need determined?
c. What relevant behaviors, if any, were noted during the observation of the student?
d. What is the relationship (impact) of that behavior to the student's academic and social functioning?
e. Are there health, developmental, or medical factors that are relevant to the student's education?
f. Do these factors impact a student's education? If so, how?
g. Do environmental, cultural, or economic factors affect the student's education?

As we discussed in Chapter 1, it is impossible to separate the assessment process from communicating the results of that assessment in writing. Much of the advice we have seen about how to make a report legally defensible is actually about how to make the *evaluation* legally defensible. The federal guidelines say nothing about what must be included in your reports but they have a lot to say about what should be true about your evaluations and therefore reflected in your report. Using your state regulations as a guide, it is essential to distinguish between what must be directly included in your reports and what must be true of your assessments. Our goal in the following section is to clarify this point.

UNDERSTAND THE DIFFERENCE BETWEEN WHAT LEGALLY MUST BE INCLUDED IN YOUR REPORTS AND WHAT MUST BE TRUE ABOUT YOUR ASSESSMENT

A distinction we often discuss in our workshops is between what must be true about your evaluations and what must be explicitly included in your reports. This distinction grew out of a conversation between one of the authors and a special education attorney who was an early collaborator on this project (J. Riel, personal communication, 2009). For what must be true about your evaluation, ultimately the evaluator should be prepared to testify to the truth and accuracy of those points. To the extent possible, these "truths" about the evaluation should be evident to the readers of your reports. In other words, you should *show* the truth of these legal mandates rather than simply *tell* the reader they are true.

Another title for this section might be "Quoting the law in your report does not make it or your evaluation more legally defensible," or perhaps even more straightforwardly, "Saying it does not make it true." Many reports we read are full of legal-sounding boilerplate language that tells the reader that the evaluation has followed legal guidelines. Often, school psychologists have a standard set of paragraphs that they cut and paste into all their reports stating that their evaluation has met all legal guidelines, as if these boilerplate statements were protective talismans that could ward off the evil questioning of attorneys and advocates. For the most part, we believe this muddles the focus of reports, making them harder to read, and does little if anything to make them more legally defensible. For example, the following statement (or something similar) regarding assessment procedure decisions is in many of the reports we read:

> *The student's primary language, ethnicity, and cultural background were taken into consideration prior to the selection of the assessment procedures. The tests chosen should be interpreted within the limits of their measured validity.*

This paragraph has two parts. One makes a claim about the evaluation process and the other offers advice to the reader. When reading the claim that the evaluator took the students' primary language, ethnicity, and cultural background into consideration prior to the selection of the assessment procedures, the first question that comes to mind is *how was this done?* In other words, what evidence supports the truth of this claim? Frequently, there is little actual evidence included in the report to support the claim. As for the validity advice, it is not clear how this would be helpful to a reader since the task of understanding validity and interpreting assessment results is the writer's responsibility, not that of the parent or teacher reading the report. In other words, the burden to choose valid assessments and interpret them accurately is on the author of the report and not the reader.

Contrast the previous boilerplate language example with information about how assessment procedure decisions were made in Marie's evaluation:

> *Marie's first language was Spanish and her mother noted that she continues to speak Spanish at home with her parents. Her academic instruction has been in English since she enrolled in Kindergarten and Marie reports she speaks English with her classmates and neighborhood friends. When asked, Marie said she believes her English skills are stronger than her Spanish skills. For this reason, Marie was interviewed in English and the tests used in this assessment were administered in English. Her cognitive abilities were assessed by tests that minimized the requirement to respond verbally to questions. Additional assessment was done in Spanish to provide further information about Marie's abilities.*

This statement is not a claim but rather an explanation of how the legal and ethical mandate to consider language and culture in the evaluation process was met. Marie's example suggests that the writer has made a reasonable good-faith effort to consider these issues in designing and conducting the evaluation. Another important difference is that this statement is about a particular child, Marie, while the first statement is generic and could be about any child. The truthfulness and accuracy of any legal claim about the evaluation process can be communicated only by information about an individual child, not by vague general statements. In contrast, the statement in the boilerplate example expects the reader to accept the statement as fact. It does not provide us with any information that allows us to judge the truthfulness of the claim. Consider also the following information, which occurred later in Marie's report:

> *As part of this evaluation, Marie was administered selected tests from the Woodcock Johnson IV Tests of Cognitive Abilities (WJ IV COG) and the Woodcock Johnson Diagnostic Supplement to the Tests of Cognitive Abilities (WJ DS). Together the WJ IV COG and the WJ DS provide two measures of general intellectual ability. One, the General Intellectual Ability–Bilingual, is a measure of intellectual ability that incorporates an assessment of oral language in English and Spanish. The second, the General Intellectual Ability–Low Verbal, does not include a measure of oral*

> *language skills but instead assesses intellectual ability with tasks that have low verbal demands.*

Although you may have made a different professional judgment about what instruments to use or not use in this case, this selection of assessment procedures seems logical given the information provided earlier in Marie's report. Taken together, the two paragraphs provide reasonable evidence for the truth of the legal claim, "The student's primary language, ethnicity, and cultural background were taken into consideration prior to the selection of the assessment procedures," rather than simply saying it was true or presenting a boilerplate statement as fact.

The second part of the boilerplate-language statement contains a statement that is not a claim but rather seems more like a reminder: "The tests chosen should be interpreted within the limits of their measured validity." As stated earlier, since the burden of interpretation is on the writer of the report, not the reader, it is not clear for whom this advice is written. In addition, it is not clear what the writer means by "measured validity," other than you should use the tests and procedures chosen for your evaluation for the purposes they were intended. Again, since it is the job of the evaluator rather than the reader to understand validity and use tests and procedures for their intended use, the statement simply confuses the reader and provides no legal confirmation that it is true.

Let us look at another commonly used boilerplate statement:

> *The tests and other assessment materials chosen for this assessment included those tailored to assess specific areas of need. No single procedure was used to determine eligibility for special education and/or determining appropriate educational programming.*

Ask yourself, "What is the author claiming?" and then, "What information would I be looking for to assess the truth of this statement?" Our guess is that the author is claiming that she conducted a comprehensive evaluation and used best practices in interpreting the data and making decisions. As we have argued, simply making a claim that something is true does not make it so. Ahead are different sections from one of our reports that, taken together, support the truth that the evaluation was comprehensive (i.e., the evaluation assessed all areas of suspected and related needs). They also demonstrate that data from multiple sources were integrated and synthesized for the reader to help support the Individualized Education

Plan (IEP) team in their decisions for special education eligibility, services, and placements. Contrast the boilerplate-language statement with the following statements from the academic section from Max's report:

Max's current academic achievement was assessed through a review of his educational records, classroom observations, teacher reports, interviews, and curriculum-based assessments. Although Max's academic skills in all areas have grown this school year, he continues to perform significantly below grade-level standards in reading, with specific weaknesses in phonics-based decoding skills.

Within the same section, we provide detailed information about Max's reading skills to help the reader better understand his academic needs. Taken together, these statements clarify the reasoning behind our assessment procedure choices and demonstrate a comprehensive approach to assessing Max's reading skills.

In October, Max's average reading fluency was assessed at 39 words per minute. The goal level for a fifth-grader would be 90–120 words per minute. As part of the general education language arts program, Max worked with his teacher in small groups three times per week for 20 minutes. The focus of these groups was increasing fluency and decoding skills. In November, Max's fluency was retested at 42 words per minute. Because of his limited progress, Max began working more intensively with the Resource Specialist Program (RSP) teacher two times per week in a small group for 30 minutes. Text rereading and sight-word memorization strategies were used to increase Max's reading fluency. With this reading intervention, Max was able to increase his fluency by 17.5 words in a 12-week time period and met his goal of increasing his reading fluency by 1.5 words per week.

TRY IT!

SHOW THAT YOUR EVALUATION HAS MET LEGAL MANDATES

Try removing the boilerplate legal language or any other generic statements from your reports. Does what remains in your report provide evidence or show that you have met the legal obligations for evaluation? What information do you need to add so that you *showed* your evaluation met legal guidelines rather than simply *told* the reader what you did?

WHAT MUST BE TRUE ABOUT YOUR EVALUATIONS (AND THEREFORE REFLECTED IN YOUR REPORTS) ACCORDING TO FEDERAL LEGAL MANDATE?

IDEA's guidelines form the legal basis for our practice. Although these guidelines do not specify what must be included in your report, IDEA has quite a bit to say about evaluations and much of this is contained in Sec. 300.304, *Evaluation Procedures* (IDEA, 2004). This section contains several important points that must be "true" about your evaluations. Remember, simply placing these statements in your report does not make them true. We have included the IDEA section 300.304 for your reference. In the remainder of the chapter, we highlight aspects of the law we believe are important to consider. We have organized these into themes, which include our recommendations of how to meet these legal mandates. These broad recommendations represent our thinking about how to approach these issues. Each of these topics is complex and could be its own book. For the sake of simplicity, we have divided these points into the following themes:

1. The evaluation should be comprehensive.
2. The evaluator should use a variety of assessment tools or approaches that gather functional and relevant data.
3. The evaluation should be fair.
4. The evaluator should be competent.
5. The procedures used should be valid and reliable.

Individuals with Disabilities Education Act (IDEA)

Sec. 300.304 Evaluation Procedures

(a) **Notice**. The public agency must provide notice to the parents of a child with a disability, in accordance with Sec. 300.503, that describes any evaluation procedures the agency proposes to conduct.

(b) **Conduct of evaluation**. In conducting the evaluation, the public agency must:

    (1) Use a variety of assessment tools and strategies to gather relevant functional, developmental, and academic information about the child, including information provided by the parent that may assist in determining:

        (i) Whether the child is a child with a disability under Sec. 300.8; and

        (ii) The content of the child's IEP, including information related to enabling the child to be involved in and progress in the general education curriculum (or for a preschool child, to participate in appropriate activities);

(2) Not use any single measure or assessment as the sole criterion for determining whether a child is a child with a disability and for determining an appropriate educational program for the child; and

(3) Use technically sound instruments that may assess the relative contribution of cognitive and behavioral factors, in addition to physical or developmental factors.

(c) **Other evaluation procedures.** Each public agency must ensure that:

(1) Assessments and other evaluation materials used to assess a child under this part:
   (i) Are selected and administered so as to not be discriminatory on a racial or cultural basis;
   (ii) Are provided and administered in the child's native language or other mode of communication and in the form most likely to yield accurate information on what the child knows and can do academically, developmentally, and functionally, unless it is clearly not feasible to so provide or administer;
   (iii) Are used for the purposes for which the assessments or measures are valid and reliable;
   (iv) Are administered by trained and knowledgeable personnel; and
   (v) Are administered in accordance with any instructions provided by the producer of the assessments.

(2) Assessments and other evaluation materials include those tailored to assess specific areas of educational need and not merely those that are designed to provide a single general intelligence quotient.

(3) Assessments are selected and administered so as to best ensure that if an assessment is administered to a child with impaired sensory, manual, or speaking skills, the assessment results accurately reflect the child's aptitude or achievement level or whatever other factors the test purports to measure, rather than reflecting the child's impaired sensory, manual, or speaking skills (unless those skills are the factors that the test purports to measure).

(4) The child is assessed in all areas related to the suspected disability, including, if appropriate, health, vision, hearing, social and emotional status, general intelligence, academic performance, communicative status, and motor abilities.

(5) Assessments of children with disabilities who transfer from one public agency to another public agency in the same school year are coordinated with those children's prior and subsequent schools, as necessary and as expeditiously as possible, consistent with Sec. 300.301(d)(2) and (e), to ensure prompt completion of full evaluations.

(6) In evaluating each child with a disability under Sec. 300.304 through 300.306, the evaluation is sufficiently comprehensive to identify all of the child's special education and related service needs, whether or not commonly linked to the disability category in which the child has been classified.

(7) Assessment tools and strategies that provide relevant information that directly assists persons in determining the educational needs of the child are provided.

THE EVALUATION SHOULD BE COMPREHENSIVE

In several places, the federal law mandates that evaluations should be comprehensive. We believe this mandate can be divided into two parts. The first part focuses on assessing in all areas of suspected disability. The second part focuses on assessing in all areas of related need.

If we are required to assess in all areas of suspected disability and need, it is in no way best practice to assess everything imaginable to cover our bases. Instead, we must first determine what disabilities and areas of need are suspected. Determining this is largely a pre-assessment activity, which then drives the evaluation process. This seems self-evident but our experience is that many psychologists do not spend the time up front to establish these hypotheses, often writing an Assessment Plan with minimal knowledge of the concerns that led to the referral.

Evidence of this can be found in reports that state the reason for referral in the broadest terms, such as, *The student was referred for an evaluation by the SST team due to academic concerns*, or by practitioners who use the same set of assessment procedures for every student, regardless of referral reason or concern. We will further discuss this in Chapter 3, though for now it is important to plant the seed that the best ways to identify suspected areas of disabilities are through (a) good communication with the referring party, be it a parent or teacher, and (b) a solid review of existing information, including the students' records, *before* the assessment plan is signed and the evaluation begins.

Legally, your obligation does not stop with suspected disabilities. We are also required to assess in all areas of related need. One way to conceptualize this is to imagine creating a list of the child's challenges and needs. Some of these needs and challenges will be directly linked to the definition of a disability and thus inform what the suspected disabilities are. Others, although part of this individual child's profile, may not be directly linked to a diagnosis or eligibility category. For example, take the disability of autism. The definition of *autism* in the federal statute is:

Autism means a developmental disability significantly affecting verbal and nonverbal communication and social interaction, generally evident before age three that adversely affects a child's educational performance. Other characteristics often associated with autism are engagement in repetitive activities and stereotyped movements, resistance to environmental change or change in daily routines, and unusual responses to sensory experiences (Assistance to States for Education of Children with Disabilities Program and the Preschool Grants for Children with Disabilities Program, 2006).

If you are assessing a child and the concerns are that he has difficulty making and keeping friends and trouble adapting to changes in routine, these would perhaps suggest autism as a possible disability. This same child might have a great deal of anxiety or difficulty attending to academic tasks. These challenges, although commonly found in children with autism, are not part of the federal or most state definitions, though they would also need to be addressed in the evaluation. The bottom line, legally and professionally, is that you are responsible to assess in *all* areas on this hypothetical list.

It is important to develop an accurate list of concerns early in the evaluation process. This provides a focus for your evaluation and informs your choice of assessment procedures. Although it is always possible to discover something about a child you did not suspect going into an evaluation, it is our experience that most often it is feasible and practical to narrow the suspected disabilities to a small number of possibilities. In essence, these become our working hypotheses about the child's disability classification. This sharpening of focus clarifies the evaluation process and prevents us from over-assessing children, making the assessment process less intrusive for children and teachers. It simultaneously saves us time and makes for a more coherent assessment. Surely this is a win-win for everyone involved.

This process of problem clarification and narrowing down of the suspected disabilities and relevant domains of need begins with parents and teachers, who are the primary source of referrals. It is our experience that the time invested early in the evaluation process clarifying consumers' concerns saves time later and prevents the assessment from being a fishing expedition in search of a disability.

There are two broad types of data available to practitioners to help them identify suspected disabilities and areas of need. One is the *hard* data of group test scores (e.g., state, district, school), academic benchmarks, office referrals for discipline violations, screenings, and so forth. Indeed, given the federal mandates for data collection and progress monitoring of academic progress across different groups of students, schools often seem awash with these types of data. Unfortunately, they are frequently underutilized.

The second type of data is the *soft* data that come from teachers, parents, and even students in the form of their perceptions of the referral concerns. These perceptions are most often communicated in their responses to interview questions or written questionnaires. Interviewing teachers and parents about their perceptions of the problems can help practitioners frame the problem and develop hypotheses about the diagnoses (i.e., What IDEA disability categories are suspected in this situation?) and areas of need (i.e., What areas of functioning are of most concern for this child, even if not part of identifying the disability?). It is beyond the scope of this book to discuss all the instruments and possible interview protocols that might assist practitioners in doing this. We have successfully used the interview guide in Appendix III with children, parents, and teachers. It reflects our bias toward developing an understanding of strengths as well as possible diagnoses and areas of need, which, while not strictly speaking a legal requirement, provides a more comprehensive picture of children's functioning.

The softer data of teacher or parent referrals are subject to the biases that arise from differing performance expectations. There is evidence that more objective data, such as *curriculum-based measurement* (CBM) or *systematic behavioral screening tools*, can help reduce bias in referrals and identify children for early intervention (Kamphaus, DiStefano, Dowdy, Eklund, & Dunn, 2010; Minneapolis Public Schools, 2001; Raines, Dever, Kamphaus, & Roach, 2012; Severson, Walker, Hope-Doolittle, Krotochwill, & Gresham, 2007). Yet, the soft data of consumers' concerns expressed in their own terms help us understand the problem in the context of a particular classroom or family. Both forms of data have value and can be helpful in assisting us in meeting the legal mandate of assessing in all areas of suspected disabilities and domains of need.

TRY IT!

IS YOUR EVALUATION COMPREHENSIVE?

1. Do you clearly identify the suspected disabilities and areas of need?
2. Are there clear data included in the Reason for Referral or background sections that show the reader how you came to suspect these particular disabilities (e.g., descriptions of symptoms or behaviors linked to the problem, discussion of performance data such as benchmarks, curriculum-based assessment data, or state or district testing, etc.)?
3. Did you assess all areas of suspected disability?
4. Did you assess in all other areas of need?

THE EVALUATOR SHOULD USE A VARIETY OF ASSESSMENT TOOLS OR APPROACHES THAT GATHER FUNCTIONAL AND RELEVANT DATA

The second theme in meeting legal assessment mandates again has two parts and focuses on (1) using a variety of means to gather data, and (2) gathering data that are both functional and relevant. The law does not provide guidance on how we might interpret *variety*, but we are certain it does not simply mean more tests. More is not always better. One way to understand what constitutes variation as part of a comprehensive assessment is the acronym *RIOT* (Leung, 1993). In this model, the mnemonic *RIOT* or (a) record review/history, (b) interviews, (c) observations, and (d) tests, guides the assessor through a comprehensive assessment by focusing on a variety of assessment procedures that provide a distinct range of information. The evaluation entails gathering and interpreting information about the student in a variety of settings and under varied conditions. Merrell suggests another rubric for judging the comprehensiveness of evaluations with the *Rule of Two* (Levitt & Merrell, 2009). Like RIOT, the Rule of Two focuses on the principle that a comprehensive assessment must have multiple elements, but as Levitt and Merrell put it, "acknowledges the reality that resources and time are often limited" (2009, p. 19). The Rule of Two suggests that a comprehensive assessment should include information from a minimum of two settings, two informants, and two assessment methods. We suggest the integration of the Rule of Two and the framework of RIOT as a way to incorporate a variety of assessment tools and data sources into your evaluation.

Besides using a variety of assessment tools, we must gather data that are both functional and relevant. The notion of *functional* is not defined in IDEA but the subsequent regulations include the following comment:

It is not necessary to include a definition of "functional" in these regulations because we believe it is a term that is generally understood to refer to skills or activities that are not considered academic or related to a child's academic achievement. Instead, "functional" is often used in the context of routine activities of everyday living. (*Federal Register*/Vol. 71, No. 156/Monday, August 14, 2006/ Rules and Regulations, p. 4661)

Given this position, we believe it is reasonable to interpret *functional* as similar to what is often described as *adaptive behaviors*. Although often used narrowly in the context of the diagnosis of intellectual disabilities, adaptive behavior is a wider construct that is important for all children. Sternberg (1985) provides another perspective on the definition of *functional* in his description of practical or contextual intelligence, which he describes as the ability to adapt to the demands of an environment. According to Sternberg (1985), *practical intelligence* "deals with the mental activity involved in attaining fit to context" (p. 45).

Adaptive behavior has been described in different ways but a consensus has emerged that it can be divided into three broad areas: (1) practical skills such as self-care, use of transportation, and so on; (2) conceptual skills such as the application of academic skills to everyday situations; and (3) social and interpersonal skills (Tassé et al., 2012). We would add two more areas to provide a fuller picture of functional skills: (4) the planning and organizational skills commonly associated with the neuropsychological construct of executive functioning; and (5) intrapersonal skills such as emotional self-regulation.

The implication of the mandate to gather functional information is clear. We must extend the focus of our evaluations beyond the purely academic and cognitive to include life skills that are related to success in all school environments, including outside of the classroom (i.e., playground, cafeteria, auditorium, etc.) and, in some cases, the home environment. Given the everyday nature of these life skills, we believe it is not sufficient to describe a child's functioning in these areas purely in terms of performance on standardized tests. We view this legal mandate as requiring us to include data about performance in the classroom, on the playground, and in the home, where functional skills would be called upon. At a minimum, we recommend that the evaluation, including the pre-referral process we describe on page 19 include a screening for these important functional skills to determine if they are potential areas of need.

We suggest the use of Table 2.1 as a way of thinking about your assessments and understanding if you have gathered functional information as part of your assessments. The table is designed to help you decide whether the assessment procedures you have chosen are providing you with functional data. Each assessment procedure is given a score from 0 to 2, representing the quality of the data the assessment procedure provides.

In Table 2.2, we provide an example of an analysis of the information collected during a learning disabilities evaluation for Lisa, a second-grade student whose main academic concern is reading and reading-related anxiety that is impacting school attendance. During this evaluation, we used the WISC-V as part of the cognitive assessment. The WISC-V data provide extensive standardized information about Lisa's overall cognitive ability and perhaps support for underlying hypotheses, though it provides no functional data regarding her reading difficulties or anxiety. The WIAT-III, a standardized achievement assessment, provides some general standardized academic data that could begin to identify areas of reading need; however, the WIAT-III was not designed as a curriculum-based assessment and Lisa's performance on this measure may not align with the reading strengths and weaknesses she demonstrates

Table 2.1   Does My Assessment Contain Functional Information About the Student's Skill?

ASSESSMENT PROCEDURE USED	PROVIDES STANDARDIZED DATA: 0 = NO OR LITTLE DATA 1 = SOME DATA 2 = EXTENSIVE DATA	PROVIDES FUNCTIONAL DATA GROUNDED IN REAL-LIFE CONTEXTS: 0 = NO OR LITTLE DATA 1 = SOME DATA 2 = EXTENSIVE DATA

Table 2.2   Does My Assessment Contain Functional Information About the Student's Skill?

ASSESSMENT PROCEDURE USED	Provides Standardized Data: 0 = no or little data 1 = some data 2 = extensive data	Provides Functional Data Grounded in Real-Life Contexts: • 0 = no or little data • 1 = some data • 2 = extensive data
Wechsler Intelligence Scale for Children–IV	2	0
Wechsler Individual Achievement Test–III	2	0
Behavior Assessment System for Children–3: Parent Rating System & Teacher Rating System	2	1–2
Curriculum-based measurement: Reading Fluency Rate	1	2
Review Open Court Unit Test Scores	1	2
Observations during a Guided Reading Group	1	2
Interview with teacher, parent, and student regarding reading skills	0	2
Interview with teacher, parent, and student regarding anxiety	0	2

in the classroom. The Behavior Assessment System for Children–3: Parent & Teacher Rating Systems provides us with standardized information regarding the parents' and teacher's perspective of Lisa's problem and adaptive behaviors, including anxiety. If this information is further used during an interview, we can gather very specific information about Lisa's anxiety, as well as potential strengths. The next two data sources we used, the CBM Reading

Fluency Rate and Open Court Unit Test scores, will provide us some comparison data with her classmates, but also with clear functional data on how Lisa is performing in the classroom with the language arts curriculum. Lastly, the observations during Guided Reading and interviews with the teacher, parent, and student will provide us with very specific functional data about both the reading skills and the impact anxiety is having on this student. The goal is not to reach a specific total or to have ratings of 2 across all assessment procedures. Rather, through integrating these multiple sources of information, we are able to meet the challenge of incorporating functional data into our evaluation.

The concept of gathering *relevant* information is more straightforward. The information we gather must be helpful in identifying educational needs and assisting those who work with the child in meeting those needs. It is important to note that although determining a disability classification or diagnosis can be helpful, it is often of limited value in identifying specific educational needs or planning interventions. For example, when a parent or teacher learns that a child has a learning disability, the diagnosis can help organize their thinking about the child but does not necessarily help in determining specific goals or strategies. We believe that to meet the letter and spirit of the law, our assessments (and the reports we write) must do two things to be relevant: (1) Help consumers better understand children and their strengths and challenges and (2) help those who work with children understand their educational and functional needs and how to better meet those needs. Table 2.3 is designed to help you determine if you have gathered *relevant* information as part of your assessment. Each assessment

Table 2.3   Does My Assessment Contain Relevant Information About the Student's Skill?

ASSESSMENT PROCEDURE USED	Helps Consumers Understand the Child Better, Including Determining a Diagnosis or Disability Classification: 0 = not helpful 1 = somewhat helpful 2 = very helpful	Helps Consumers Work More Effectively with This Child. Directly Leads to Interventions and/or Accommodations: 0 = not helpful 1 = somewhat helpful 2 = very helpful

procedure is given a score from 0 to 2, representing the relevance of the data the procedure provides. There is no specific number we are trying to achieve when using this table. The table simply helps us reflect on our evaluation and ensure we have used a variety of data sources and have gathered relevant data.

In Table 2.4, we take the example of Lisa's assessment further to review the relevance of the collected data. Using our standardized and functional data, Lisa was identified as having weak phonics-based decoding skills. Although we could probably identify this concern with data from the standardized measures used, such as the Wechsler Individual Achievement Test–III and the Comprehensive Test of Phonological Processing, neither of these measures is precise enough to provide the relevant data needed to write academic goals or create interventions. Think about the results you get from a standardized achievement test. Is a standard score from an index or subtest, such as, *Lisa's score on the Word Reading subtest was 88*, enough information to write a quality IEP goal or help the teacher create an intervention? No, it is not. Through the use of curriculum-based tools, such as a district-created phonemic awareness test, we can identify specific phonemic awareness or phonics-based decoding skills that Lisa is missing, such as consonant sounds, long vowel sounds, short vowel sounds,

Table 2.4   Does My Assessment Contain Relevant Information About the Student's Skill?

ASSESSMENT PROCEDURE USED	Helps Consumers Understand the Child Better, Including Determining a Diagnosis or Disability Classification: 0 = not helpful 1 = somewhat helpful 2 = very helpful	Helps Consumers Work with This Child. Directly Leads to Interventions and/or Accommodations: 0 = not helpful 1 = somewhat helpful 2 = very helpful
Wechsler Individual Achievement Test–III	2	1
Comprehensive Test of Phonological Processing	2	1
Curriculum-based assessment, such as School District Phonemic Awareness Benchmark	2	2

consonant blends, sound blending, segmenting, syllabication, rhyming, and so forth. These relevant data can help us write a clear and measurable goal as well as give us insight into appropriate interventions.

THE EVALUATION SHOULD BE FAIR

Assessment should be designed to yield the best results for a child. Specifically, the law says two things: The tools used as part of the assessment (1) should not be racially or culturally biased and (2) should be chosen to yield accurate information about a child, given the child's language and culture but also limitations in his or her sensory (vision and hearing), motor, and speaking skills.

Although the mandate that the assessment be fair is clear, the process of how one does this is less straightforward. Much of the literature has focused on the complicated issue of fairness in the assessment of bilingual and bicultural youth (e.g., Figueroa & Newsome, 2006; Lau & Blatchey, 2009; Olvera & Gomez-Cerrillo, 2011; Ortiz, 2008; Ortiz, Flanagan, & Dynda, 2008; Rhodes, Ochoa, & Ortiz, 2005). Two models of how to approach this issue systematically have been developed by Olvera and Gomez-Cerrillo (2011) and Rhodes, Ochoa, and Ortiz (2005). Olvera and Gomez-Cerrillo's MODEL approach (2011) shares many of the attributes we discussed in the section on how to ensure assessments are comprehensive. *MODEL* stands for (a) multiple sources of information, (b) observation, (c) data-driven hypothesis, (d) English-language development, and (e) language of assessment. Like RIOT (Leung, 1993), MODEL gives practitioners guidance on how to judge the comprehensiveness of an assessment, but does this in the context of working with bilingual and bicultural youth.

Ochoa and Ortiz's (2005) model helps practitioners determine the best language(s) to use in the assessment to yield the most accurate results. They recommend that practitioners consider: (a) the grade of student; (b) the mode of assessment (i.e., reduced culture and language "load," native language, English, or both languages); (c) the current and previous types of educational program (e.g., native language, bilingual education, sheltered English, pullout English-language development, etc.); and (d) the child's proficiency in both English and the native language (Rhodes, Ochoa, & Ortiz, 2005, p. 169).

In terms of making your assessments and the reports you write legally defensible, regardless of the model you use, it is important for practitioners to document a systematic process by which they have determined the fairest way to approach an assessment. Rather than making the unsupported generic boilerplate statements we discussed earlier in the chapter, reports should provide specific information about how these decisions were made for a particular child in a specific context.

The following are examples of what this might look like in reports. We do not believe they are perfect but rather demonstrate a good-faith effort to make our thinking about evaluation fairness transparent to the reader.

Examples: Demonstrating Fairness in Your Evaluation

Phuong's parents are from Vietnam and they speak mostly Vietnamese at home. He is in the fifth grade and has received instruction in English since preschool. During the assessment, Phuong always spoke in English, even when addressed in Vietnamese. He was talkative but sometimes difficult to understand because he spoke softly and made frequent errors in pronunciation. Phuong mostly spoke in single words, short phrases, or simple sentences. Because of this, his academic skills were assessed in English but his intellectual abilities were assessed by tests that provide basic and simple English verbal instructions and that do not require verbal responses.

~

Tanya's first language was Spanish. She speaks Spanish with her mother and a mix of English and Spanish with her friends and neighbors. All of Tanya's academic instruction has been in English and when she was administered the Woodcock Language Proficiency Battery–Revised, her language skills were significantly stronger in English than they were in Spanish. When asked, Tanya said that she thought she understood and spoke English better than Spanish. For these reasons, the assessment was conducted in English with occasional Spanish prompts and translation when needed.

~

José is a third-grade student at Jones Elementary. His native language is Spanish and he speaks mostly Spanish at home. At school, José speaks Spanish with his Spanish-speaking peers and English with his teacher. His communication with his English-speaking classmates is limited. José was educated in El Salvador from Kindergarten through second grade. He is currently classified as an English-language learner (ELL). In addition to a California English Language Development Test (CELDT) level of Early Intermediate (Listening and Speaking), José also

---

> *demonstrated an English Cognitive Academic Language Proficiency Level (CALP)*
> *of 1, suggesting his oral English skills are minimal and he would have difficulty*
> *understanding classroom instruction in English. His CALP level in Spanish is a 4*
> *(Woodcock Munoz Bateria). Given that he appears to have stronger language skills*
> *in Spanish and has been mostly educated in Spanish, his cognitive and academic*
> *skills were assessed in Spanish.*

These three examples do two important things. They provide information about the child's language development and pattern of language usage and offer a rationale for how the assessor considered the issue of fairness in the assessment. For an English-speaking child with limited verbal abilities or impaired hearing or vision, the logic would be similar. For example, note the rationale for fairness used here for an English-speaking 10-year-old child with high-functioning autism:

> *When Randy's cognitive abilities were previously assessed using the Wechsler*
> *Intelligence Scale for Children, his performance was mixed, with scores rang-*
> *ing from high average to far below average. His strongest performance was*
> *on tasks of visual perception and problem solving and he had most difficulty with*
> *tasks that involved verbal expression and verbal memory. Given this pattern, as*
> *part of the current evaluation Randy was given the Kaufman Assessment Battery*
> *for Children Non-verbal Index (KABC Non-verbal Index). The Non-verbal Index*
> *consists of five different tests of cognitive ability that all emphasize visual reason-*
> *ing or problem solving. Taken together, these tests provide an estimate of cog-*
> *nitive functioning for children who have difficulty understanding or using oral*
> *language. Randy's performance on the KABC Non-verbal Index was above aver-*
> *age for students his age.*

The issue of fairness is a complicated one and there are several ways to consider it in your assessments and write about it in your reports. This section is not meant to be a comprehensive treatment of the issue and, though the previous statements each have their limitations, they all represent efforts to make the authors' thinking transparent to the reader. In other words, they try to *show* rather than just tell the reader that the evaluation was fair.

THE EVALUATOR SHOULD BE COMPETENT

How can someone make a legal judgment regarding your competence? There is no professional or official consensus for a legal standard of expertise, although several attributes can be taken into consideration. These include: (a) years of experience; (b) accreditations (e.g., licenses, certificates, etc.); (c) peer identification (i.e., Is this person well known in the field?); (d) between-experts reliability (i.e., Are this person's judgments similar to other experts?); (e) within-person reliability (i.e., Are this person's judgments reliable over time?); (f) subject matter expertise (i.e., using an acknowledged "super-expert" as a reference point); and (g) factual knowledge (e.g., how well you can respond to questions) (Shanteau, Weiss, Thomas, & Pounds, 2003).

Considering these attributes, we believe there are two general answers to how our competence is judged. One is professional experience and the other is scope of practice. Professional experience incorporates years of experience and knowledge of types of assessment and assessment tools. Professional experience also can encompass experience with a particular population, including special education eligibility categories, mental health or medical diagnoses, school placements, ethnicity, or socioeconomic status. In general, it represents our acquired experience. For example, both of us are competent in all areas of school psychology (i.e., basic expertise in our scope of practice), yet Michael has extensive experience with mental health problems and assessment related to the special education category of Emotional Disturbance. In contrast, Jeanne Anne has considerable experience with children from diverse cultural and socioeconomic backgrounds, the disability category of Autism, and the functional assessment of academic skills. In a legal context, all of our experiences would bolster the argument for general competence and expertise in specific areas.

The second aspect of legal competence is scope of practice and is reflected by our qualifications, licenses, and certifications. School psychologists' range of practice can be broad. We can be engaged in psychoeducational evaluations, suicide or threat assessments, parent–teacher consultations, group counseling, and providing professional development. It is common for some of us to participate in all of these activities in the course of a day. Our scope of practice is directly related to, but not limited by, our professional experience. All school psychologists must meet state certification requirements to practice in the schools, though many school psychologists have extra certifications, licenses, or trainings that expand their scope of practice.

We think it is important to review the scope of practice of school psychologists because we often have conversations with practitioners where they have set artificial limits on their ability to address problems in the schools. These include things like, "We can't identify children with that because it is a medical diagnosis," or "You have to be licensed as a therapist or clinical psychologist to provide that service." Of course, we should always practice within our experience and training, but it is also important to know that in schools our roles are broadly defined to include a wide range of skills and services. For example, the National Association of School Psychologists (NASP) describes the work of school psychologists thus:

School psychologists help children and youth succeed academically, socially, behaviorally, and emotionally. They collaborate with educators, parents, and other professionals to create safe, healthy, and supportive learning environments that strengthen connections between home, school, and the community for all students. (National Association of School Psychologists, n.d.)

The NASP Blue Print III (2006) goes on to define four *functional competencies* that school psychologists should have:

1. Data-based decision making and accountability
2. Systems-based service delivery
3. Enhancing the development of cognitive and academic skills
4. Enhancing the development of wellness, social skills, mental health, and life competencies

These competencies are a required part of the training students receive in any NASP-approved graduate program. We can assume from the breadth of these standards that the national organization that represents school psychologists and determines our ethical standards sees the scope of practice as including systems and individuals as well as encompassing cognitive, academic, and social-emotional development.

Scope of practice will differ somewhat from state to state but will have similarities. For example, in the California Education Code, school psychologists and their services are described in Section 49424:

A school psychologist is a credentialed professional whose primary objective is the application of scientific principles of learning and behavior to ameliorate school-related problems and to facilitate the learning and development of children in the public schools of California. To accomplish this objective the school psychologist provides services to children, teachers, parents, community agencies, and the school system itself. These services include:

a. Consultation with school administrators concerning appropriate learning objectives for children, planning of developmental and remedial programs for pupils in regular and special school programs, and the development of educational experimentation and evaluation.

b. Consultation with teachers in the development and implementation of classroom methods and procedures designed to facilitate pupil learning and to overcome learning and behavior disorders.

c. Consultation with parents to assist in understanding the learning and adjustment processes of children.

d. Consultation with community agencies, such as probation departments, mental health clinics, and welfare departments, concerning pupils who are being served by such community agencies.

e. Consultation and supervision of pupil personnel services workers.

f. Psychoeducational assessment and diagnosis of specific learning and behavioral disabilities, including, but not limited to, case study evaluation, recommendations for remediation or placement, and periodic reevaluation of such children.

g. Psychological counseling of and other therapeutic techniques with children and parents, including parent education.

We have reviewed several other states' descriptions of what services school psychologists provide and it is clear that, like California, their scope of practice allows them to provide a wide range of evaluation, consultation, and treatment services in schools. There is no doubt that when it comes to assessment for special education purposes, school psychologists would be judged as legally competent.

THE PROCEDURES USED SHOULD BE VALID AND RELIABLE

The final theme involves using assessment procedures that are both valid and reliable. Validity and reliability are complex issues and it often intimidates school psychologists when they find out that the requirement to use valid and reliable measures falls on them. In other words, it is our responsibility to establish whether a tool we are using is valid and reliable. It is not the responsibility of our school district, which may very well purchase and own tools that do not meet the standards for validity and reliability described in the American Psychological Association's (APA) *Standards for Educational and Psychological Testing* (American Educational Research Association [AERA], APA, & National Council on Measurement in Education, 2013).

We will begin with reliability, because a test cannot be valid if it is not reliable. Reliability refers to the consistency of a measure. Does the measure provide stable results when the testing procedure is repeated? For example, if a test is designed to measure cognitive ability, then each time the test is administered to a student, the results should be approximately the same. We use the word *approximately*, because even under standardized conditions, variations in performance are going to be reflected in the student's scores on the measure.

We call this *measurement error*. Measurement error is the difference between a student's observed or obtained score and his or her hypothetical "true" score. Reliability provides a measure of the extent to which an examinee's score on a test reflects random measurement error.

When a student is given a standardized measure, measurement error is caused by factors specific to the student (e.g., motivation, hunger, fatigue), factors specific to the test or measure (e.g., unclear directions, poor choice discrimination), and factors specific to scoring (e.g., vague scoring criteria, computational errors). In a more reliable test, these errors are minimalized, though they cannot be eliminated. In a less reliable test, a child's performance can vary significantly and thus be less dependable, especially when making high-stakes decisions (e.g., does this score represent evidence of a significant weakness, suggesting a disability?). Lastly, composite and index scores are often more reliable (i.e., have less measurement error) than individual subtest scores, which is why interpretation at the subtest level can be inappropriate.

In the end, it is our responsibility to choose and use reliable measures (remember, not the readers of your reports!). Fortunately, reliability evidence for standardized measures typically can be found in the test manual (consider it a red flag if you cannot find it!). This allows us, as practitioners, to compare measures and choose appropriate instruments.

According to the Standards for Educational and Psychological Testing, when scores are to be interpreted and, we would add, described in a report, relevant reliability and measurement error should also be reported. We believe using confidence intervals instead of reporting obtained single scores is an easy-to-understand approach to conveying this information (e.g., not "Rina earned a 100" but rather "There is a 90% chance that Rina's score falls between 90 and 110"). Confidence intervals are an estimated range or band of scores that contain the obtained score plus or minus a margin of error. Test manuals routinely provide information on confidence intervals at the 68%, 90%, and 95% levels. For example, when a 95% confidence interval is used, we are providing a statement of reliability that we are 95% sure that the student's true score falls within this range of scores (AERA, APA, National Council on Measurement in Education, 2013). There are, of course, different arguments to be made for different levels of confidence, but we have generally settled on 90% as a minimal level of acceptance.

For a test to be valid, evidence and theory need to support or demonstrate a relationship between the test and the behavior it is reported to measure. Valid measures are effective because they provide accurate information on the construct the measure was designed to assess. Simply put, validity is the extent to which a test measures what it says it measures. For example, when getting a driver's license, the formal driving test given through the Department of Motor Vehicles is probably a more valid measure of your actual ability to drive on city streets than the written test that is also given. Conversely, the written test may be a more valid measure of your knowledge of your state's driving laws than the formal driving test. Unfortunately, the concept of validity is not as clear in psychological testing.

Validity is an important concept because it is fundamental to appropriate test interpretation. Test performance must be interpreted within the construct the test proposes to assess. Many test developers provide claims of validity in their manuals, though they do not provide evidence to support that their measure is more valid than another method for gathering similar information. For example, a standardized test of written language ability might focus on having students write complete sentences in response to prompts. This test does not measure the ability to compose a multi-paragraph essay, or use persuasive language in writing, which we could argue are equally valid aspects of the construct of written language ability.

Test interpretation is also influenced by extraneous circumstances that are not related to the measure itself or the construct assessed. Perhaps the student had an emotional response to the writing prompt, the testing environment was loud, the student misunderstood the directions, or the evaluator made an error in test administration. In summary, validation is the mutual responsibility of both the test developer and the test user. The test developer should present evidence that his or her measure is appropriate for its intended use. The test user is responsible for evaluating the test developer's claims and then using and interpreting the test correctly.

In this chapter, we have reviewed the federal guidelines set forth by IDEA and the subsequent regulations regarding the legal aspects of assessment and report writing. Unfortunately, most of the legal guidelines for assessment are stated very generally. We are left to define many of these mandates ourselves. In this chapter, we have tried to provide brief descriptions of best practice to draw upon to fill in these blanks. One of the takeaway messages is that there is no great separation between best practices and the notion of legal defensibility. Another important message from this chapter is that our reports serve as evidence that we have met the legal obligations of our evaluations. The critical word is *evidence*. It is not enough to tell the reader that we have met these legal mandates but we are obligated to *show* the reader how this was accomplished.

It is our view that the answer to how to make a report legally defensible is to conduct an assessment that is fair and comprehensive and uses a variety of procedures designed to gather functional and relevant information, so we can respond directly to the concerns raised by the parents and teachers who initiated the assessment. In the following chapter, we will answer the question, "How do I make my reports more useful to consumers?" We will introduce the concept of *useful* and review our main strategies for how to make your reports more understandable and accessible for consumers, specifically parents and teachers.

Chapter 2 Takeaway Points

- A legally defensible assessment and report incorporates legal mandates with best practices.
- Using your state regulations as a guide, it is essential to distinguish between *what must be directly included* in your reports and *what must be true* of your assessments.
- To meet IDEA legal mandates:
  - The evaluation should be comprehensive.
  - The evaluator should use a variety of assessment tools or approaches that gather functional and relevant data.
  - The evaluation should be fair.
  - The evaluator should be competent.
  - The procedures used should be valid and reliable.
- Good practice and the spirit of the law suggest that parents (and all IEP members) should be given copies of all reports before a meeting so they have the time to read and thoughtfully consider this information.
- Our reports serve as evidence that we have met the legal obligations of our evaluations. The critical word is *evidence*. It is not enough to tell the reader that we have met these legal mandates but we are obligated to *show* the reader how this was accomplished.
- Quoting the law in your report does not make it or your evaluation more legally defensible.
- Remove the boilerplate legal language or any other generic statements from your reports. Make sure you *showed* your evaluation met legal guidelines rather than simply *told* the reader it did.
- To meet the letter and spirit of the law, our assessments and reports must do two things to be useful: (1) Help consumers better understand children and their strengths and challenges and (2) help those who work with children understand their educational and functional needs and how to better meet those needs.

How Do I Make My Reports More Useful to Consumers?

In Chapter 2 we reviewed the legal mandates for reports and evaluations. In Chapter 3, we focus on the concept of usefulness, including why focusing on making our reports more useful should be a major goal of our writing. We will outline our recommendations for how to make reports more useful for consumers, specifically parents and teachers. In doing this, we build on the research literature touched on in Chapter 1 as well the ethical standards of our profession. As a reminder, thus far we have highlighted that our reports should address specific referral concerns and help those who work with children to do their jobs better. In essence, useful reports support these two themes.

Research indicates that consumers characterize useful psychoeducational reports as clear and understandable. For example, understandable reports communicate assessment data using language that is easily understood by the consumer (Harvey, 1997, 2006; Rafoth & Richmond, 1983; Weddig, 1984). Useful reports also clearly answer the referral questions, focus on strengths as well as needs, and provide concrete and feasible recommendations for educational planning (Brenner, 2003; Cornwall, 1990; Eberst & Genshaft, 1984; Teglasi, 1983; Wiener, 1985, 1987; Wiener & Kohler, 1986).

These assumptions of report accessibility and usefulness are reflected in the ethical guidelines of both national school psychology professional organizations. NASP's *Principles for Professional Ethics* (NASP, 2010) and the American Psychological Association's (APA) *Standards for Educational and Psychological Testing* (American Educational Research Association [AERA], APA, National Council on Measurement in Education, 2013) maintain that assessment findings should be presented in language clearly understood by the recipients and the report should support the recipients in their work or interactions with the child.

Write Your Report with the Audience in Mind

In order to thoroughly examine the concept of usefulness we need to consider our audience or the report consumers. Although often considered a type of technical writing, we believe that psychological reports are best conceptualized as stories. In this, they share with other stories a need for a clear plot that pulls the reader along and characters, both main and supporting, who despite their flaws are portrayed in the most accurate and positive light possible. Often stories are complicated, as are children, but it is our job to pull the threads together to communicate a comprehensive view of the child and come to specific conclusions. Beyond a clear plot, the structure and language you use to tell a story will depend on your audience. Given this, the first question we then must ask ourselves about our reports is: *Who is our intended audience?*

Many individuals, including parents, school administrators, outside professionals, and sometimes legal counsel, read assessment reports hoping to better understand a child's cognitive, academic, emotional, or behavioral functioning. However, we strongly argue that the most important consumers of a psychoeducational report are the student's parents and teachers. Teachers and parents usually initiate psychoeducational assessments and implement the assessment recommendations (Gilman & Medway, 2007). If our reports are designed to positively influence their interactions with students and assist with educational planning, school psychologists need to know how to make the information in written reports more useful and understandable for these critical consumers.

Physicians most often write to other physicians, and attorneys most often write to other attorneys. This allows them to use a shared vocabulary and style that is designed to communicate information in an economical and helpful fashion to insiders. This makes their writing efficient for a specific audience but also makes these communications nearly impossible to decipher by those outside these professions. Psychoeducational reports are different in that they are in large part intended for consumers outside of the psychological profession, including, most importantly, teachers and parents. Unfortunately, many reports appear to be written with the wrong audience in mind. Given the amount of boilerplate legal language and technical psychological jargon used, perhaps many school psychologists are writing for other school psychologists or attorneys with a background in special education law. These reports often become compliance documents that are very difficult to read, rather than useful communication tools.

This is not a problem unique to school psychology, nor is it a new phenomenon. In Tallent and Reiss's 1959 survey of over 700 Veterans Administration mental health workers, the greatest criticism of psychological reports was that they were not written "with a useful purpose in mind" (Tallent & Reiss, 1959, p. 444). This problem persists despite a consensus in the literature that useful reports: (a) are understandable by the consumer, (b) provide specific answers to individualized referral questions, (c) focus on strengths as well as needs, and (d) give specific and feasible recommendations (Brenner, 2003; Cornwall, 1990; Eberst & Genshaft, 1984; Teglasi, 1983; Wiener, 1985, 1987; Wiener & Costaris, 2012; Wiener & Kohler, 1986). To return to our story metaphor, they tell a story to a particular audience, offer a balanced depiction of the protagonist, and come to a concrete conclusion. In the following sections we will explore each one of these characteristics in detail.

USEFUL REPORTS CLEARLY ANSWER THE REFERRAL QUESTIONS

In Chapter 1, we defined *assessment* as the process of gathering information to inform decisions. This process involves collecting and evaluating data for the purpose of responding to stakeholders' questions and concerns, identifying needs and strengths, and making meaningful recommendations. Perhaps we should have clarified that this is the definition of a *useful* assessment. To be perceived as useful, we believe that an assessment and corresponding report have to directly respond to the concerns of parents and teachers.

It makes intuitive sense that a psychoeducational evaluation would be designed to answer the questions posed by those who referred the child. However, more often than not, we see assessments that are designed around a protocol of assessments geared toward a specific disability classification. For example, *all* students suspected of having a learning disability are assessed using Test A, Test B, Test C, and Test D, regardless of individual differences, strengths, or concerns. Although this system of assessment may gather lots of data, it may not be useful or helpful in supporting those who live and work with the child to better understand the child's needs. Since a primary goal of a useful report is to answer the referral questions, we must identify these questions early in the evaluation process. We can then design our assessment to gather specific data to answer the referral questions and then clearly answer these questions in our report.

To develop these questions, we recommend two strategies. First, we recommend a thorough review of records, including an examination of cumulative school records and work samples. Understanding the child's educational history and progress will help identify suspected areas of disability and need. Second, collaboratively create the assessment plan with the parents, teachers, and other service providers requesting the evaluation. This can take place at a meeting with all parties present or through individual conversations with each person. Through these two steps, you will clarify the concerns to be addressed in your assessment and identify suspected areas of disability and need. As reviewed in Chapter 2, this facilitates meeting the legal mandate of conducting a comprehensive assessment. In Chapter 4 we will review how to write referral questions and use those questions and answers as a structure for your report.

Useful Reports Focus on Strengths as Well as Needs

Addressing strengths as well as problems and pathology has become a common recommendation in psychology and related professions (Snyder, Ritschel, Rand, & Berg, 2006). In addition, there is considerable support for addressing strengths in reports (Brenner, 2003; Brown-Chidsey & Steege, 2005; Cornwall, 1990; Eberst & Genshaft, 1984; Teglasi 1983; Wiener, 1985, 1987; Wiener & Costaris, 2012; Wiener & Kohler, 1986). Philosophically we strongly support this approach and in our own practice we have attempted to integrate a strengths perspective into our evaluations and the reports we write. As Snyder and his colleagues explain, "Each individual exists and functions in a variety of contexts by using a combination of strengths and weaknesses" (2006, p. 34). To be comprehensive, we believe that it is important to account for the full range of a child's functioning and not just focus on challenges and problems.

Including strengths and resources in a comprehensive evaluation has several advantages. Conversations about strengths encourage greater participation in the assessment process and subsequent interventions (Epstein, Hertzog, & Reid, 2001). They encourage practitioners to focus on the enhancement of skills and learning while simultaneously reducing problems or symptoms (Epstein et al., 2001; Nickerson, 2007).

Integrating client strengths into your evaluation can be accomplished by working closely with the referral sources to formulate referral questions that consider assets and strengths as well as problems (Snyder, Ritschel, Rand, & Berg, 2006). In addition, it is important to incorporate a schema for how to consider strengths into our understanding of our assessments. In addition to the models of RIOT and the *Rule of Two* (Leung, 1993; Levitt & Merrell, 2009), discussed in Chapter 2, Snyder et al. (2006) have suggested a four-level matrix that guides practitioners to assess for both assets and weaknesses within the client and the environment (Snyder & Elliott, 2005; Wright & Fletcher, 1982). This matrix can help guide our assessment questions and the data we collect, as well as the themes that we develop from our assessment results. In essence, the matrix simply encourages you to include the student's personal and environmental assets as well as challenges.

In the following example, Max is a newly assessed fifth-grader who will soon be transitioning to middle school on a new campus. His psychoeducational report may be his first

Table 3.1   Incorporating Strengths as Well as Needs into an Evaluation

Environmental Assets	Environmental Challenges
Personal Assets	Personal Challenges

introduction to his new teachers, so a goal is to clearly discuss his learning disability and our recommendations in the report. But it is equally important that the report reflects Max's strengths as well as his weaknesses. In this example, information about his personal assets helps the reader understand that although Max reads at a mid-third-grade level, he is very intelligent and mature for his age.

Example: Including Student Strengths in Your Report

> *Max demonstrates many behaviors and skills that are consistent with average to above-average cognitive ability. Max is proficient with grade-level math computation and applied problems. Max demonstrates leadership qualities in non-academic areas and has well-developed social skills with peers and adults. He resolves conflict thoughtfully and logically. Max is able to engage in age-level conversations with peers and adults. He gives appropriate and sequential explanations and is able to describe non-academic interests and experiences with detail. He shows creativity in stories told and questions asked. Max has strong listening comprehension skills. He remembers information and facts, from stories read to the class as well as movies and television programs he has watched at home. Max also demonstrates a clever sense of humor and understands jokes that many of his peers do not yet completely grasp.*

Later in the report, his strengths were used to write the following recommendation:

> *Max has demonstrated excellent leadership skills and is well liked by other students. Encouraging Max to join clubs and/or sports teams in middle school will help to continue his success with his peers and provide him with positive leadership opportunities.*

USEFUL REPORTS PROVIDE CONCRETE AND FEASIBLE RECOMMENDATIONS FOR EDUCATIONAL PLANNING

Results from several studies suggest that consumers such as teachers and parents have a very practical view of reports. Although they might find our results and diagnostic conclusions interesting and perhaps useful, they are most concerned about the implications of these conclusions and our recommendations. Many reports lack meaningful recommendations, either because the results do not actually lend themselves to practical recommendation or the authors have avoided offering recommendations out of what we believe is an incorrect fear that they will legally bind the team to accept their recommendations and provide the services implied by their suggestions.

In their report writing guide, Wolber and Carne (2002) assert that individualized and pre-scriptive recommendations are the hallmark of a useful report. Research has supported their claim. As early as 1945, Cason argued that reports utilizing vague generalizations and lack-ing appropriate and specific recommendations hindered communication between teachers and psychologists (Cason, 1945). In 1964, Mussman conducted an informal evaluation of report content with a small group of teachers. The teachers surveyed placed high value on the recommendation section. Brandt and Giebink (1968) corroborated Mussman's findings. In their investigation of experienced elementary and high school teachers, they found that reports with specific recommendations were preferred over reports with abstract recom-mendations. Hagborg and Aiello-Coultier (1994) evaluated teachers' perceptions of psycho-educational reports they received on their students. The vast majority of the teachers rated themselves as satisfied to very satisfied with the school psychologist's report. However, teachers also indicated they viewed the report as an opportunity to receive specific sug-gestions and strategies and that the recommendations provided were often too few and too abstract. These findings were consistent with the results of Davidson and Simmons' (1991) qualitative survey of special and general education teachers, and special education teach-ers in training. The respondents in this study maintained that much of the information in reports was irrelevant to their work with students. They saw a need for a more collaborative approach to the assessment, use of classroom terminology and constructs, and clear recom-mendations for intervention.

Parents have also identified clear and individualized recommendations as a highly valued assessment outcome. In their study, Tidwell and Wetter (1978) had parents complete a ques-tionnaire designed to determine their expectations and satisfaction with their child's psycho-educational evaluation. The participants identified the recommendations and suggestions for helping them work with their child as the primary motivation for the evaluation and the most valued part of the psychoeducational report.

Consider the following recommendation, which is required to be included in all reports by a school district near us: *Share and discuss evaluation results with the IEP team and discuss appro-priate educational interventions.* What is remarkable, given the research showing that useful recommendations are what consumers value the most in reports, is that this is the only rec-ommendation provided. Consider this from the perspective of a worried parent or teacher waiting for some information that will help them understand and help a child. You have spent several hours assessing the child, they have waited at least a few weeks and up to two months to get the results, and in the end, you essentially have nothing to recommend other than the fact that the IEP members should read your report and then talk about it. This is not useful and, at a minimum, would be incredibly frustrating for many of the IEP team members. A neurologist colleague of ours likens this to diagnosing someone with a seizure disorder with the only recommendation being that the patient discusses this with his general practitioner (J. Donnelly, personal communication, 2012).

It is clear that, legally, a "group of qualified individuals" including the parent establish eligibility for special education services and, if needed, develop an Individualized Education Plan (IEP). However, this does not imply that the person or persons who conducted the assessment should not make meaningful recommendations that contribute to the IEP or, if the child is not eligible for special education services, make appropriate and helpful recommendations to the general education teacher or parents. Indeed, we have to ask ourselves why anyone would value our services if, in the end, we have nothing useful to say about the child we have assessed.

The avoidance of making meaningful recommendations seems a solution in search of a problem. We have been told that this type of generic pass-the-buck non-recommendation is a precautionary measure so that the school district will not be obligated to provide whatever an evaluator recommends. This is incorrect and legally there is no obligation to provide what an evaluator recommends (McBride, Dumont, & Willis, 2011). There is an obligation to consider the recommendations provided in evaluation reports, though it is up to the IEP team to decide what services and accommodations are appropriate to be placed in the IEP. Indeed, there is an ethical aspect to providing useful recommendations. For example, the 1997 version of the ethical standards of the National Association of School Psychologists was very clear that there is an ethical obligation to write reports that "assist the student or client" and "emphasize recommendations and interpretations" (National Association of School Psychologists, 1997, p. 29). In the most recent NASP *Principles for Professional Ethics* (2010), it is implied throughout the Professional Competence and Responsibility standards that recommendations are a responsibility of the school psychologists' practice.

A positive perception of the usefulness of reports by teachers has also been shown to increase the likelihood that recommendations stemming from a psychoeducational evaluation are followed (Andrews & Gutkin, 1994; Gilman & Medway, 2007). Interestingly, and as a segue to our next theme, in their evaluation of the persuasiveness of psychoeducational reports, Andrews and Gutkin (1994) demonstrated that increasing text understanding, familiarity, and message quality within a report were factors that enhanced report influence and increased teacher compliance with recommendations. In other words, clear and understandable writing can impact teachers' consideration and cooperation with your recommendations. We will cover writing good recommendations in Chapter 4, but for now, remember teachers and parents place high value on recommendations that are detailed and appropriate for implementation in the school environment (Bagnato, 1980; Mussman, 1964; Salvagno & Teglasi, 1987).

Here are a few examples. These recommendations are linked to the assessment results, are student specific, and reflect an understanding of the classroom environment and curriculum.

Examples: Include Useful Recommendations in Your Report

Anthony has made significant academic progress and is meeting many grade-level standards. He is currently successfully mainstreamed into a general education second grade for 90 minutes a day of language arts instruction. Anthony has demonstrated good work habits and motivation and the IEP team needs to consider further mainstreaming during core subjects. His continued need for placement in a special day class should be reviewed by his IEP team before he transitions to third grade.

Abigail can currently read and spell the first 200 sight-words from the Frye sight-word list. Continued flashcard practice for 10 minutes each day with the next 200 words will improve her fluency and accuracy in both reading and writing.

Valerie has gaps in her phonemic awareness and poorly developed phonics-based decoding skills. Remediation needs to focus on re-teaching the phonics-based reading program. She needs direct instruction in short- and long-vowel sounds, decoding long- and short-vowel patterns, consonant blends (i.e., bl, sl, tr, cr,), and diagraphs (i.e., st, sh, ch, th) to increase her decoding skills and reading fluency. When interviewed about her reading skills, she did not appear to have a solid understanding of where her strengths and weaknesses are. Valerie was surprised to see how many words she could read. It was explained to her that she is good at memorizing words, though not figuring out unknown words. Valerie's strengths and challenges should be thoroughly reviewed with her so she is clear on what aspects of her reading she needs to work on.

USEFUL REPORTS ARE CLEAR AND UNDERSTANDABLE

Making the information from psychological assessments accessible or understandable to consumers is important for practical, legal, and ethical reasons. The National Assessment of Adult Literacy (United States Department of Education, 2003) assessed English literacy levels of over 19,000 adults representing the entire population of U.S. adults, 16 years of age and older. NAAL classified participants' literacy levels into five descriptive categories. Adults categorized as non-literate possessed no literacy skills. Adults in the Below Basic category were described as having the most simple and concrete literacy skills with the ability to locate easily identifiable information in short, commonplace text. Basic categorization implied that adults could perform simple and everyday literacy activities, such as reading and understanding information in short common text. Intermediate and Proficient levels were described as performing moderately to complex literacy activities such as reading, summarizing, making inferences, and synthesizing text. Based on their data collection, the NAAL concluded that the prose literacy skills for 43% and the quantitative literacy skills for 55% of the adult population in this country were at a basic level or below.

The results of the NAAL survey have ethical and legal implications for report writing. At least half the adult population (and we are certain this is a very conservative estimate) does not possess the literacy skills to read and comprehend the information provided in a typical psychoeducational report. Not only is this counterintuitive if parents are among the main consumers of our reports, but it can be argued that this violates their rights under IDEA (Harvey, 1997; Weddig, 1984).

IDEA (2004) provides clear guidelines regarding parents' right to be involved in the evaluation process and to participate in the decisions that follow. Yet, to involve parents in this process authentically, they must have access to adequate information that is understandable, which is one of the key tenets of informed consent (Lidz, 2006). If parents cannot read or understand the psychoeducational report, they cannot be informed participants in their child's educational planning and decision making (Weddig, 1984). One barrier to this is that often the written information contained in reports is communicated in a way that few parents can understand. The ethical and legal obligation to ensure that parents have access to the information they need to authentically and fully participate in the evaluation and decision-making process falls on us as professionals.

READABILITY IMPACTS THE USEFULNESS OF YOUR REPORTS

One of the most important ways of making the information in psychological reports more understandable is to increase the readability of the text. *Readability* is a term associated with the ease of reading proficiency and comprehension of written material. Reader competence, level of education, and word and sentence difficulty are factors that are correlated with the readability and comprehension of text (Klare, 1976). There are several ways to determine readability but most formulas use a combination of vocabulary and sentence complexity to calculate how easy it is to read a passage or document. Formulas such as the Flesch-Kincaid Grade Level and the Flesch Reading Ease have been used since the mid-1930s to provide information on the amount of formal schooling needed to read and comprehend text (Flesch, 1948; Klare, 1976).

Readability is important because researchers going back several decades have consistently found that increasing the readability of text such as a magazine or newspaper article, through using simpler vocabulary and sentence structures, both increased the number of people who actually read the material and improved the comprehension of those readers (Lostutter, 1947; Murphy, 1947; Schramm, 1947; Swanson, 1948). Later, Klare and colleagues found that improving readability increased both the amount read and the amount learned among Air Force recruits (Klare, Mabry, & Gustafson, 1955; Klare, Shuford, & Nichols, 1957). It is interesting to note that Lostutter (1947) found that the reading ease of newspaper articles had little to do with the education level of the writer but rather reflected the conventions and culture of the newspaper industry. This implies that perhaps psychological reports are not written at a graduate level because the authors have advanced degrees and knowledge, but rather they are following the conventions of the profession.

Here is one of our favorite examples of this concept in action: Klopfer (1960), an early report writing researcher, wrote, "It is my contention that any statement found in psychological reports could be made comprehensible to any literate individual of at least average intelligence." This sentence has a Flesch-Kincaid Reading Level of 17.8, meaning that a graduate education level would be needed to read and understand this statement with ease. No offense to Dr. Klopfer, but by using simpler vocabulary and sentence structure, this sentence can be rewritten to "I think a psychological report can be written so most people can understand it." This sentence now has a Flesch-Kincaid Reading Level of 9.2, meaning a typical high school freshman could read this sentence with ease. The content of the sentence is still intact; it is just presented in much more understandable language.

Despite the advantages of increasing the readability of reports, most research has found that a very high level of literacy skills is needed to comprehend the average psychological report. For example, in Weddig's (1984) analysis of traditional psychological reports, the mean readability was at the 14.5-grade level. Several years later, Harvey (1997) found similar readability levels and suggested that school psychology graduate students receive direct training in how to make their written reports more accessible for the reader.

Almost 20 years later, Harvey provided the same suggestion in her exploratory study of the variables affecting report clarity and understanding (2006). Harvey evaluated the language usage within psychological report examples and models collected from 20 textbooks commonly used for training school psychology graduate students. Ironically, the majority of textbooks recommended writing clear and understandable reports, though they provided sample excerpts and reports with a mean Flesch-Kincaid Reading Level calculated at 18.5.

We believe that reports can be written in such a way as to increase their readability and enhance their accessibility for parents and teachers. For example, in Weddig's (1984) research, a traditional psychological report written at the 15th-grade level was rewritten at a 6th-grade level by replacing professional terminology with behavioral descriptions and eliminating information considered irrelevant to educational decision making. Parents reading the modified (i.e., 6th-grade level) report scored significantly higher on a comprehension test than those reading the traditional report (i.e., 15th-grade level). This finding supports the recommendation that lowering the readability level of psychological reports will facilitate parental understanding while maintaining adequate coverage and validity of the assessment information.

TRY IT!

WHAT IS YOUR READABILITY LEVEL?

Check your readability level. We think you may be surprised at the results.

1. Pick one of your typical psychoeducational reports and estimate what readability level you think it is written at.
2. Run the Spelling and Grammar check on the document in your word processing program, and when the correction box pops up enter the Options function, then check the box to show your readability statistics. Once you have completed the Spelling and Grammar check for the document, your readability statistics will pop up.
3. Are you shocked? We were, the first time we did this!
4. The following link provides further information about Microsoft's readability statistics: http://office.microsoft.com/en-us/word-help/test-your-document-s-readability-HP010148506.aspx.

Increasing the readability of reports is helpful for all consumers but especially critical for parents who may not have the literacy skills for or familiarity with the psychological language we use in our reports. This is not an easy task and there is no goal readability level that we set. Both of us have actively worked on increasing our report readability. On average, we write reports at approximately an 11th- to 12th-grade Flesch-Kincaid Reading Level (FKRL). We both strive to lower our FKRLs further with a goal of approximately 9th to 10th grade. So, how do we actually do this? We provide four suggestions to help increase the readability level of your written reports. First, reduce the professional or technical jargon. Second, cut extraneous words and use an active voice. Third, carefully consider the length, including amount and quality of information included in your reports. Fourth, use a report structure that integrates data and highlights relevant assessment findings.

INCREASE READABILITY BY REDUCING PROFESSIONAL JARGON

Psychological jargon or the use of technical terminology in reports has been frequently identified as a hindrance to understanding by both psychologists and non-psychologists (Harvey, 2006; Ownby, 1997; Tallent, 1993; Weddig 1984). It is a common recommendation in books and guidelines on report writing to avoid jargon or technical terms if you can.

Although the language used within written reports can be controlled and altered by the writer, the lack of consensus among school psychology practitioners and test publishers regarding technical terms such as *working memory, auditory processing,* or *learning disabled* makes this task a formidable one (Harvey, 2006; Rafoth & Richmond, 1983). For example, in her survey of practicing psychologists, Harvey (2006) requested a narrative and numerical definition of the term *average intelligence.* The results suggested that the participating psychologists did not have a standard definition for the term, noting that 30% of respondents disagreed with the most commonly used numerical definition and provided qualitatively different narrative definitions. Rafoth and Richmond (1983) investigated the level of understanding and perceived usefulness of psychological terms by school psychology students, education students, and practicing special education teachers. Although educators with a special education background rated some technical language as more useful, in general, disagreement was noted in the usefulness of some frequently used terms such as *hyperactive, grade level,* and *developmental delay.*

In many of our workshops we ask the participants to define a technical term often seen in psychoeducational reports, such as *visual processing.* Although scientific rigor in this task is clearly absent, the results have been the same in dozens of trainings. The participants struggle with this activity. They usually stop making direct eye contact with us, perhaps in fear we may call on them to answer the question. Rarely do we have a participant who wants to share his definition in front of a large group of his professional peers. What are the implications for these findings, both the research based and our anecdotal? Perhaps, as a field we do not have a professional consensus on what many of these technical terms mean. This dilemma will hopefully lead us to question our belief that these terms have an unambiguous meaning and that they are somehow self-explanatory for the reader of our report.

We recommend that you be cautious in using this kind of language, and when you need to use technical language, make sure to explain each term in the context of the student and evaluation. Rewrite technical information using easily understood language and vocabulary and provide clear behavioral examples when using technical terms. If this seems a formidable task for you, remember it will be no easier for the reader. Put simply, if you cannot clearly define a term or provide examples of what it looks like, we recommend that you do not use it.

Consider the following examples of John and Kelly, two Kindergarteners. The technical jargon is presented, and then rewritten using the recommendation to rewrite technical information using easily understood language and providing clear behavioral examples. As a side note, ask yourself which description is more helpful. Which description provides information for the IEP team to make decisions about services, goals, and accommodations?

Examples: Rewriting Technical Jargon

Rewrite technical information using easily understood language and provide clear behavioral examples:

Technical jargon: John's visual-motor integration is in the average range.

John's visual-motor skills are developing normally. When copying line drawings, John used proper pencil grip and braced the paper when drawing. He knew when he made a mistake and asked to redo two of his drawings. His letter formation has continued to improve and he now legibly writes all upper- and lowercase letters. In the classroom, John's penmanship is best when he is given lined paper for boundaries and reminded to concentrate and do his best work. When writing in his journal, John uses the word wall in his classroom. Either sitting at his desk or using a clipboard from the floor, he is able to accurately copy words from the wall, letter by letter. During whole-group language arts lessons, John is also able to follow and simultaneously complete written assignments his teacher is modeling from an overhead projector.

Technical jargon: Phonological awareness is the knowledge of the sound structure of the English language. It is the ability to hear and manipulate units of sound, such as onsets, rimes, and syllables. Kelly's phonological awareness skills are below average.

Phonological awareness helps children learn how letters and sounds go together in language that supports learning to read and write. It includes understanding

(continued)

> (*continued*)
>
> *that words are made up of sounds represented by letters. It also includes the ability to manipulate sounds by identifying rhymes* (bat/cat) *and words that start or end with the same sounds* (bat/ball; cat/rot), *dividing words into smaller parts, such as syllables and sounds* (table = *ta/ble*), *blending separate sounds into words* (b/e/d = bed), *and adding, deleting, or substituting sounds in words* (c/a/p − a + u = c/u/p).

INCREASE THE READABILITY OF PSYCHOEDUCATIONAL REPORTS BY CUTTING WORDS AND USING ACTIVE VOICE

Although it is perhaps unusual to cite George Orwell in a book written for psychologists, Orwell's advice on writing is useful. In his essay, *Shooting an elephant and other essays* (1950), Orwell proposed six rules for writing. We paraphrase four of them that we think are especially useful for authors of reports:

1. Never use a long word when you can use a short one instead.
2. If it is possible to cut a word out, cut it out.
3. Never use the passive voice where you can use the active voice.
4. Never use a scientific word or jargon if you can think of an everyday English equivalent.

Numbers 1 and 4 relate to our discussion of professional jargon. Numbers 2 and 3 can also go a long way toward making your writing more readable. Cutting words is easy once you develop an eye for it. Some examples are small. For example, why say "school context" or "preschool setting" when "school" or "preschool" will do just as well? Other examples involve cutting the unnecessary language out of sentences. Consider this sentence:

John has not experienced any significant changes related to his health and development in recent years.

That's not a terrible sentence, but we can easily cut words and make it clearer:

John has not had any significant changes in his health in recent years.

Or, better yet, use positive phrasing and say:

John is healthy.

Notice that we have gone from 16 words to 3. If John's health was actually poor and there had been no changes, we, of course, would have phrased this differently. But, most of the time, writers are simply referring to a health status that is unremarkable in the sense that the child is healthy and has no significant health or medical problems. In that case, "John is healthy" will almost always work just fine.

Here is a 33-word sentence:

John demonstrated satisfactory progress in all areas of personal growth and study habits, with the exception of "completes and returns homework on time," in which he received a grade of E (excellent progress).

One revision could reduce this to 31 words, which is not a big savings:

John earned grades of "satisfactory progress" in all areas of study habits on his report card except "completes and returns homework on time," where he earned a grade of "excellent progress."

But if we consider the essential meaning of this sentence, we could say:

John earned grades of "satisfactory" to "excellent progress" in all areas of study habits on his latest report card.

Another way to cut words in reports is to remember Steven King's writing adage: "The road to Hell is paved by adverbs" (King, 2000). Adverbs and adjectives are sometimes referred to as "intensifiers" and are used when you think the reader needs an extra boost to get your point. If Stephen King can get by without adverbs writing horror fiction, then writers of psychological reports can get by without them, too.

Passive voice is when the object of an active sentence (I interviewed John) is made into the subject (John was interviewed). Too much passive voice will deaden your writing and make it harder to read. We acknowledge that passive voice is difficult to avoid in psychoeducational reports, especially when you make the choice to not use the personal pronouns *I* or *me*. The question is one of degree. Use passive voice sparingly and avoid it when you can. An example of a sentence written in passive voice that could be easily changed to active voice is:

In the preschool setting, John's difficulty with managing anger, frustration, and fear was noted.

The first question is, who noted these behaviors? In this case let's assume it was the teachers. The conversion to active voice would be:

In preschool, John's teachers observed that he had difficulty managing anger, frustration, and fear.

Note that we also removed "setting," which is an example of cutting unnecessary words. We include two more examples to really drive the point home:

Passive: **His behavior at school is similar at home, according to John's parents.**
Active: **John's parents said his behavior at school is similar to home.**
Passive: **John was adopted at birth.**
Active: **Mr. and Mrs. Lopez adopted John at birth.**

Although we prefer active voice, we will opt for passive voice instead of referring to ourselves in the third person such as "this psychologist" or "the interviewer." To the average reader of our reports, this will simply seem odd. For us, it seems too clinical. We are writing the report for an audience. "I" conducted the assessment and wrote the report, so it seems peculiar to refer to myself in the third person as "the psychologist." However, if you are part of a multidisciplinary assessment and report, simply use active voice when clarifying who conducted each part of the evaluation. Our final example provides an idea of what these might look like:

Passive voice, third person: **John was observed during recess by the school psychologist.**
Active voice, third person: **The school psychologist observed John at recess.**
Active voice, first person: **I observed John at recess.**

You can use your word processing software to help reduce passive voice. Most word processing programs allow you to set the spelling and grammar function to check the percentage of sentences written in a passive voice. When running a spelling and grammar check, the grammar function will highlight the passive sentences and the readability statistics we reviewed earlier will provide a percentage of sentences. Again, there is no perfect percentage, but we have set personal goals to have 20% or fewer passive sentences in our reports.

TRY IT!

CONVERT PASSIVE VOICE TO ACTIVE VOICE

Check the readability statistics of your report and then set the review function of your word processing software to detect passive voice. See how many of your passive voice sentences you can change to an active phrasing. Recheck your readability statistics. What difference did it make?

INCREASE THE READABILITY OF PSYCHOEDUCATIONAL REPORTS BY CONSIDERING THE LENGTH, INCLUDING AMOUNT AND QUALITY OF INFORMATION

As we noted in Chapter 1, we have observed a trend in the area where we practice toward very long reports of 30-plus pages. Reports of this length can be difficult to read for anyone, let alone parents and teachers. Interestingly, some of the research on readability we discussed earlier in this chapter found that a newspaper story nine paragraphs long lost 3 out of 10 readers by the fifth paragraph, making a case for shorter rather than longer reports (Lostutter, 1947). Lengthy reports often have considerable generic, rather than individualized information about the actual child being assessed, and include a level of detail that is rarely helpful to consumers. Another problem we have observed is that these long reports do not integrate or interpret information in a way that is easy to follow, thus lacking a coherent plot and breaking the first rule of a good story. In addition to our own observations, several researchers have found that longer reports are not preferred or considered more useful than shorter ones (Brenner, 2003; Brown-Chidsey & Steege, 2005; Donders, 1999).

There is no magic number of pages for reports, and both children and evaluations vary in their complexity. Research on the preferences of both parents and teachers suggests that integration of information and recommendations, not report length, are most important (Wiener, 1985, 1987; Wiener & Kohler, 1986). Both of us have done many complex evaluations with children that have had significant referral concerns, often involving information from multiple sources. It is a rarity that these reports have exceeded 20 pages, a number that strikes us as probably longer than necessary. On average, we write reports between 5 and 10 pages. Some have suggested that once reports become longer than five to seven pages, the length may become a barrier to understanding the information (Weiner, personal communication cited in Mastoras, Climie, McCrimmon, & Schwean, 2011). Our own experience bears this out. Although we are obviously sophisticated readers of reports, we often lose patience with longer reports and find ourselves flipping through the pages searching for a summary or some concise presentation of what is meaningful.

Report length is sometimes a function of adding unnecessary detail about every aspect of the evaluation. This "throwing data on a page" obscures our primary task as assessors, which is to make meaning of the data gathered and communicate this meaning in a way that is helpful. Part of what makes this information difficult to understand is that it is not really about the child being assessed but rather consists of generic language, often cut and pasted from test manuals, that does not communicate anything meaningful to the readers of the report. Another problem is that scores and observations are often described in great technical detail, which unfortunately can obscure what the data actually mean for those who work with a child.

The research finding that integration of information is a key consumer preference also suggests that much of the generic technical information and boilerplate claims about the legality of your evaluation could be easily left out of reports or, in some cases, placed in an appendix at the end of the report. This would serve to both shorten most reports and place the focus of the report on the student-specific data and information presented. A simple recommendation is, to the maximum extent possible, focus the content of a report on the specific child assessed. This seems like a straightforward point, but frequently we have found ourselves wading through large amounts of generic material in reports that could have been written about any child. We have both read independent educational evaluation (IEE) reports on students that were over 250 pages in length. In these reports, the vast majority of the information presented has nothing to do with the student who was assessed. There are pages of generic information about every assessment tool, including technical information about each subtest. Readers would literally have to weed through pages of random information to get to a sentence or two about the child and then somehow remember that information as they wade through the next 20 or so pages. This shock-and-awe method of presentation is clearly an extreme example, though it highlights the need for us to keep our audience in mind and focus on the essential information. Consider the following example, pulled directly from a report from a local school district, where Leslie's performance on the Test of Auditory Processing–3 was presented. Read this example, and then try to answer the questions that follow.

Example: Data's Meaning Lost in the Presentation

The *Test of Auditory Processing Skills, Third Edition* (TAPS-3) is an individually administered assessment of auditory processing. The test provides an overall score, Overall Auditory Processing, and three cluster scores, including Basic Auditory Skills, Auditory Memory, and Auditory Cohesion. The cluster scores are reported as standard scores with an average range of 85–115 and the subtest scores are reported as scaled scores with an average range of 7–13.

CLUSTER/SUBTEST	SCORE	QUALITATIVE DESCRIPTION
Basic Auditory Skills	**92**	**Average**
Word Discrimination	7	
Phonological Segmentation	7	
Phonological Blending	11	
Auditory Memory	**85**	**Average**
Number Memory Forward	7	
Number Memory Reversed	7	
Word Memory	8	
Sentence Memory	7	
Auditory Cohesion**	**93****	**Average****
Auditory Comprehension	5	
Auditory Reasoning	12	
Overall Auditory Processing*	**90***	**Average***

Leslie's Basic Auditory Skill cluster score of 92 fell within the average range. She scored within the average range on the Word Discrimination subtest, which assessed her ability to determine if two verbally presented words are the same or

(continued)

(*continued*)

different. She scored within the average range on the Phonological Segmentation subtest as well, which assessed her ability to manipulate syllables and phonemes within words. Leslie also performed within the average range on the Phonological Blending subtest, which assessed her ability to synthesize a word given the individual phonemic sounds (e.g., /s/a/t/ = sat). This was a relative strength for Leslie.

Leslie's Auditory Memory cluster score of 85 fell in the average range. She performed in the average range on the Number Memory Forward subtest in which she listened to a sequence of numbers and had to repeat them as she heard them. She also performed in the average range on the Number Memory Reversed subtest, in which she listened to a sequence of numbers and had to repeat them backwards. Leslie performed within the average range on the Word Memory subtest, which required her to listen to a sequence of unrelated words and repeat them as she heard them. She performed in the average range on the Sentence Memory subtest, which assessed her ability to recall a sentence from memory.

**Leslie's Auditory Cohesion cluster score of 93 fell within the average range; however, due to her range of scores this score may not be a good representation of Leslie's ability and it is important to examine her individual strengths and weaknesses. She performed below the average range on the Auditory Comprehension subtest, in which she listened to a sentence or two and was asked a question about something that had been directly stated in the sentence. This was an area of weakness for Leslie. She performed within the average range on the Auditory Reasoning, which assessed her ability to understand implied meanings, make inferences, or come to logical conclusions when given information. Auditory Reasoning subtest is specifically designed to tap auditory cohesion, a higher-order process. This was an area of relative strength for her. *Leslie's Overall Auditory Processing score of 90 fell within the average range; however, due to her range of index scores this score may not be a good representation of Leslie's overall ability and it is important to examine her individual strengths and weaknesses.

Ask Yourself:

- Are these data interpreted in a way that consumers can understand?
- Are there data from multiple sources?
- Will this information help the IEP team write goals and accommodations?

If you answered "No" to any of the questions (and we hope you answered "No" to all of them), then you have remembered some fundamentals of this book: Interpretation and integration of data is the psychologist's job, not the reader's, and our report is the foundation for the IEP team's decision making. The previous example is a classic illustration of the meaning of evaluation data being lost in the presentation. There are many reasons for this, including overuse of technical language and jargon, inclusion of unnecessary information, exclusion of any meaningful interpretation of the evaluation results, and poorly structured information and formatting. The responsibility for interpretation and integration falls on the school psychologist. In the following example, we present the same data but link performance on the standardized measure to classroom and home.

Example: Data Interpreted and Integrated

Leslie's auditory processing skills were evaluated using standardized tests, classroom observations, and interviews with her parents and teacher. Leslie's performance on the Test of Auditory Processing Skills (TAPS) was in the average range. For example, during testing, she was proficient at determining if two words she heard were the same or different, manipulating syllables and sounds in words, blending sounds together, and listening to and repeating lists of numbers and words. She also did well listening to and repeating sentences and listening to short stories and answering questions.

Interviews with her teacher and observations of Leslie in the classroom during whole-class Language Arts instruction suggest that her performance on the TAPS is consistent with the skills she uses in the classroom. Leslie demonstrates a solid understanding of lecture material. She asks relevant questions and follows along and participates actively in class discussions. At home, her parents say that she is a good listener and completes tasks correctly and quickly when asked. The family enjoys watching movies together, and based on their discussions, they believe that Leslie has good listening comprehension.

This rewrite interprets the test results in the context of all the evaluation data, without over-interpreting single-index scores (a topic for another book altogether), providing meaningful information for the reader. In doing this it also shortens the presentation from 465 words at a 13.3 FKRL to 196 words at a 12.1 FKRL.

Of course, other psychologists, special education teachers, administrators, and perhaps attorneys will also read our reports. In some cases, people who have a more extensive knowledge of evaluation will want access to technical information regarding the instruments we have used or the scores we reference. However, it is important to remember that these people are not our primary audience, so rather than make this kind of detailed technical information the focus of our reports we recommend that you be prepared to answer these questions, if asked, or perhaps place the information in appendixes or attachments at the end of your report.

Increase the Readability of Your Report by Using a Report Structure That Integrates Data and Highlights Relevant Evaluation Findings

As we demonstrated in Leslie's example, one of our major concerns about many of the reports we read is that the data are not integrated in a way that the reader can clearly understand the major findings or "big ideas." To return to our analogy of reports as stories, the plot points are unclear. In the next section, we discuss the advantages and disadvantages of different report models and propose a question-driven, theme-based report model as the most efficient report writing structure for focusing your writing on the important assessment elements and facilitating the integration of assessment data.

Report writing structures or models refer to the organizational style used to present assessment results. Like the chapters and subheading of a book or article, the structure of a report can contribute to a clear and understandable presentation of the results by guiding the readers' thinking (Ownby, 1997; Tallent, 1976; Wiener, 1987). To establish which report writing models have been traditionally taught, we reviewed common graduate school assessment training texts (e.g., Flanagan & Harrison, 2005; Salvia & Ysseldyke, 2001; Sattler, 1992, 2001, 2008) and report writing guides (e.g., Bradley-Johnson & Johnson, 2006; Lichtenberger, Mather, Kaufman, & Kaufman, 2004; Ownby, 1997, Tallent, 1993; Wolber & Carne, 2002).

Report writing is the culmination of the assessment process; however, in our review, the majority of assessment texts did not mention report writing and only Sattler (1992, 2001, 2008) devoted an entire chapter to report writing strategies. Sattler (2008) did not recommend a specific report format, though he strongly recommended assessment findings be synthesized and clearly presented. A well-written report requires the writer to integrate and analyze the assessment data. All of the reviewed guides recommended using an organizational structure to support an integrated and cohesive report. Based on our review, we have grouped report writing models into (a) test-based, (b) domain-based, and (c) referral-based.

Test-based reports are characterized by a sequenced presentation of each assessment tool (usually standardized tests) and typically use test titles as headings. The test's purpose and the student's quantitative test results are the primary information provided. In Sattler's (1992) opinion, test-based reports are the most common and the easiest to write for novice report writers because the reports often lack the more difficult-to-write qualitative interpretive information. The difficulty with a test-based report is that a well-written report requires the writer to integrate and analyze the assessment data, not simply report test performance data. Teglasi's (1983) statement that "tests do not tell the results; rather, the psychologist reports the results after using the tests to arrive at interpretation, conclusions, and recommendations" (p. 472) highlights why using a test-based structure has been discouraged by many authors (e.g., Ownby, 1997; Tallent, 1993; Wolber & Carne, 2002), including ourselves. If standardized assessment is an integral part of your assessment, then test scores may clearly be valuable. However, test scores alone are not useful, and separate from the assessor's interpretation, can be misleading for many report consumers. Presenting scores and score descriptors alone, for example, the TAPS-3 narrative earlier in this chapter lacks interpretation and leaves the process of integrating what these test data mean to the reader.

Domain-based reports present evaluation data in specific assessment categories such as Cognitive Abilities, Academic Achievement, and Social–Emotional Functioning. A pattern of strengths and weaknesses is often presented under each domain. Traditionally, the summary is the section that integrates the report sections into a whole. Many authors classify domain-based reports as a traditional report writing model for school psychologists (Batsche, 1983; Ross-Reynolds, 1990). In their most recently published guide to report writing, Bradley-Johnson and Johnson (2006) used domain-based reports as the model and exemplar. Although others' styles were reviewed, the psychological report examples by two sets of authors (i.e., Lichtenberger, Mather, Kaufman, & Kaufman, 2004; Ownby, 1997) were entirely domain based.

We acknowledge that a domain-based structure is preferable to a test-based structure, though we do not recommend the use of a domain-based model for two reasons. First, the reader often has to wade through pages of information prior to receiving key information or a summary. This can leave the reader to reconstruct the report domains into a whole. Often we see school psychologists use the headings of a domain-based report, but then revert to a test-based presentation under each domain heading. Second, in domain-based reports, the categories or domains can predetermine the areas of importance, which can make the evaluation and report less focused on unique concerns and needs.

Referral-based reports are organized around assessment-based answers to specific referral questions. Referral-based reports are a product of a referral-based evaluation where report writing is integrated into the assessment process. Assessment tools are chosen and assessment data are interpreted in the context of the referral questions and then presented by statements or thematic headings within the report. The conceptualization of a psychological assessment

Table 3.2   If Your Headings Look Like This . . .

REPORT HEADING	REPORT STRUCTURE
Woodcock Johnson IV: Test of Cognitive Abilities	Test-Based
Cognitive Ability	Domain-Based

Cognitive Ability
    Woodcock Johnson IV: Test of Cognitive Abilities
    Kaufman Brief Intelligence Test–2
	Domain/Test-Based

What are Michael's cognitive strengths and weaknesses and how do they impact his ability to access the grade-level curriculum?	Referral-Based

as a consultation-based inquiry focused on answering specific referral questions is a fundamental shift from the traditional idea of an evaluation as a search for disability or profile of students' strengths and weaknesses. If you are unsure what types of reports you are writing, Table 3.2 will help you identify the style based on the headings you are using.

Unfortunately, research investigating effective report writing models has been limited, with the majority of the literature focused on professional opinions of best practice (e.g., Lichtenberger, Mather, Kaufman, & Kaufman, 2004; Ownby, 1997; Tallent, 1993; Wolber & Carne, 2002); however, there have been a small number of studies that consider the impact of different report formats.

Mussman (1964) conducted the first published research investigating different report structures. A brief handwritten report containing a statement of the referral question, a description of the student's performance, and recommendations related to the referral question was compared to a more traditional typewritten report containing information regarding the behavior and appearance of the student during the evaluation, test scores and analyses, student interview information, and recommendations. Twenty-five teachers read a number of reports from one of the formats and then completed an opinion questionnaire regarding the reports they read. Although the study suffered from several limitations, Mussman (1964) encouraged school psychologists to self-evaluate the usefulness of their report-writing techniques.

Bagnato (1980) hypothesized that the report format and synthesis of assessment information would influence teachers' ability to match assessment information to appropriate classroom-based intervention goals. Preschool-level special education teachers read two different report formats and were asked to make judgments on appropriate educational goals.

Both reports presented the assessment information. The translated report included a thorough description of how the assessment data were linked to classroom objectives, while the traditional report did not include linkages to classroom-based practices. The teachers who received the translated report were significantly more accurate in linking the assessment information to curriculum goals than the teachers who received the traditional report. Bagnato (1980) recommended that the report writer synthesize the comprehensive assessment data, and then organize and present the information around functional domains (i.e., domain-based) rather than the test given (test-based). Bagnato also recommended that strengths and skill deficits be presented in clear behavioral terms to facilitate the creation of individualized objectives. Lastly, Bagnato recommended the inclusion of detailed educational and behavioral recommendations. These report attributes were viewed as more relevant to intervention planning and creation of individualized education goals.

Wiener (1985, 1987) and Wiener and Kohler (1986) investigated the comprehension of parents, elementary and secondary school teachers, and school administrators for different psychological report formats. Over the course of these investigations, the researchers randomly assigned participants to read one of three report formats. The Short Form was a single-page report including the reason for referral, assessment results, and succinct recommendations. The Psychoeducational Report format was a domain-based report with information clustered under specific headings. The report was written in behavioral terms with the sources of information clearly identified. Technical terminology was avoided or clearly defined and recommendations were specific and carefully explained. The Question-and-Answer report utilized a referral-based format, including the same information, terminology, and recommendations as contained in the Psychoeducational Report, though the Reason for Referral section was comprised of a list of referral questions drawn from interviews with teachers and parents. Each question was directly addressed within the report. The researchers found that the educators and parents comprehended and preferred the Psychoeducational and Question-and-Answer formats over the Short Form report. Wiener (1987) hypothesized that the domain- and referral-based reports were more coherent, facilitating connections between the assessment information presented and the readers' prior knowledge. Wiener recommended that school psychologists include clear and specific examples of technical terms and concepts, as well as elaborate descriptions of the student's current functioning and recommendations.

Salvagno and Teglasi (1987) examined the perceived helpfulness of a test-based versus an observation-based psychoeducational report. Although the teachers' ratings of helpfulness were not significantly different for the two report formats, interpretive information was consistently rated as more helpful than test-based quantitative statements. Teachers preferred interpretations that reflected the school psychologists' integration and synthesis of the assessment data and recommendations that were specific and easily implemented by the teacher.

Most recently, Carriere, Kennedy, and Hass (2013) investigated teacher comprehension and usefulness of different report structures. Teachers were randomly assigned to read a test-based, domain-based, or referral-based report, and then completed a questionnaire about their understanding of the report content, as well as their beliefs regarding the usefulness of the report itself. The results confirmed that the report writing model impacted teachers' comprehension of the information in the psychoeducational report. Report models emphasizing the integration of assessment data resulted in the highest comprehension scores, with teachers who read the referral-based report having significantly higher comprehension of report data than those who read the test-based report.

Although limited, our review of the research suggests that there is a distinct pattern of preferences by educators and parents. Parents and educators prefer reports that synthesize and integrate the comprehensive assessment data (Salvagno & Teglasi, 1987; Wiener, 1985, 1987; Wiener & Kohler, 1986). Information presented around specific areas of functioning and written in behavioral terms was preferred over a test-based presentation of information (Bagnato, 1980; Carriere, Kennedy, & Hass, 2013). Teachers also placed high value on recommendations that are detailed and appropriate for implementation in the schools (Bagnato, 1980; Mussman, 1964; Salvagno & Teglasi, 1987).

Referral-Based Reports Synthesize Fundamental Research Findings with Best Practice

At this point, it will not come as a shock that we both strongly believe a referral-based or question-driven theme-based report is the most useful and effective model. We teach and practice this model because we believe that it is the best way for us to write useful and legally defensible reports. We both see our report writing as a work in progress and neither of us believes that our reports are perfect. In fact, we read each other's reports and often have lively discussions about how to make them better. Yet, we both read and write a lot of reports and we do our best to practice what we preach. It was our commitment to making this vital part of school psychological practice more useful for parents and teachers, and our audiences' and students' enthusiasm for our trainings and workshops that led us to write this book.

We credit Batsche (1983) with developing a report writing structure that combines the fundamental research findings with best practice. His report writing model is geared toward enhancing the collaborative process between the school psychologist and the referring person. Batsche's Referral-Based Consultative Assessment/Report Writing Model was designed to clarify and answer specific referral questions through a consultative process with the referring person. These referral questions drive the assessment process, including data collection, report writing, recommendations, and intervention planning (Batsche, 1983; Ross-Reynolds, 1990). The Batsche model consists of six steps: (1) reviewing existing data on the student, (2) consultation with the referring person, (3) collaborative development of referral questions, (4) selection of assessment procedures validated to answer the referral questions, (5) integration of assessment data to answer the referral questions, and (6) developing recommendations in response to the assessment results. These steps not only guide the assessment process, but they are reflected throughout the structure of the written report.

This report model synthesizes the guidelines and recommendations we present in this book and aligns with NASP's Blueprint for Training and Practice III, which advocates that assessment activities be directly connected to prevention and intervention and focused on enhancing students' academic and social-emotional competencies (NASP, 2006). We value collaborative consultation, integrated data-based decision making, and linking assessment to prevention and intervention. We believe this aligns well with the needs and preferences of consumers; clear answers to referral questions and recommendations are exemplified in this report writing model. In Chapter 4, we go step-by-step through a referral-based report structure, explaining how to frame both your evaluation and report using this model.

Chapter 3 Takeaway Points

- We believe the most important consumers of a psychoeducational report are the student's parents and teachers. Teachers and parents usually initiate psychoeducational assessments and implement the assessment recommendations.
- If our evaluations are designed to positively influence teachers' and parents' interactions with students and assist with educational planning, we need to know how to make the information in written reports more useful and understandable for these critical consumers.
- Useful reports clearly answer the referral questions.
- Useful reports focus on strengths as well as needs.
- Useful reports provide concrete and feasible recommendations for educational planning.
- Useful reports are clear and understandable.
- Increase the readability of your reports by reducing professional jargon, cutting excess words and writing in an active voice, considering the amount and quality of information, and using a report structure that integrates data and highlights relevant evaluation findings.
- Referral-based reports are a product of a referral-based evaluation where report writing is integrated into the assessment process. Assessment tools are chosen and assessment data are interpreted and integrated in the context of the referral questions and then presented by statements or thematic headings within the report.

Step-by-Step, How Do I Write Useful and Legally Defensible Reports?

In the prior chapters, we have made a case, hopefully a convincing one, for showing rather than telling readers you have met legal mandates, making reports more useful for the consumers, and why we advocate for the use of a referral-based, question-driven format that integrates data and responds directly to consumers' concerns. In this chapter, we will examine each section of our proposed referral-based report and discuss step-by-step how to write a report using this structure. Where needed, we will discuss how this differs from what you might see in traditional test-by-test or domain-driven reports. There are several examples of full reports in Appendix II. It may be helpful for you to review some of these prior to reading how to structure a referral-based, question-driven report.

As we proceed, we want to remind you of several strategies, introduced in Chapter 3, that are overarching and perhaps not directly connected to the format you use to write your reports. These include using simpler language and reducing jargon, reducing boilerplate or generic statements, and carefully considering the level of detail needed to communicate with your intended audience.

HOW DO I CLEARLY COMMUNICATE THE PURPOSE OF THE EVALUATION?

The Reason for Referral section of the report communicates the background and rationale for the evaluation. In other words, the reader should know from reading the Reason for Referral section what led to the request for an evaluation and what issues are of concern to those who made the request. Many reports we read provide brief statements that at best point you in a general direction. They are often generic and provide little information about *this* child and *this* evaluation.

Examples: Poorly Written Reason-for-Referral Statements

A psychoeducational assessment was requested by a parent in writing on 9-1-13 due to concerns about Amy's social-emotional functioning.

A psychoeducational assessment was completed due to Mrs. Rodriguez's concerns about Carlos needing more services than those provided by his 504 Plan.

A psychoeducational assessment was completed as part of a triennial review.

A psychoeducational assessment was requested by the SST due to concerns with delays in Christy's academic progress.

These brief statements provide a vague rationale for the evaluation but communicate almost nothing to the reader about the nature of the "concerns," difficulties with academic progress," or "services" in question. In the case of "A psychoeducational assessment was completed as part of a triennial review," the author is stating a fact, which is evident in the report that follows, instead of providing an actual rationale. Of course, triennial reviews are required, but this is a generic legal requirement that communicates nothing about the particular child being reevaluated. Another example is a kind of fill-in-the-blanks template used for all evaluations in some school districts.

The purpose of this initial assessment is to determine if NAME is eligible for special education placement and/or related services. The assessment results shall be shared with the Individualized Education Program (IEP) team to enable the team to decide if NAME demonstrates one or more impairments and, if so, if the degree of the impairments requires special education and/or related services. If the IEP team determines that NAME's impairment requires special education and/or related services, the assessment results will be used to discuss NAME's unique needs and develop an appropriate IEP based on his needs. If the IEP team determines that NAME does not require special education or related services, the assessment results will be shared with the IEP team to discuss how NAME can be educated in the general education program with or without modifications.

Based on the relevant information that has been made available to the district to date, it is suspected that NAME has one or more impairments in the areas(s) of: LIST IMPAIRMENTS. This assessment examines suspected impairments in these areas. Data will be obtained from concurrent assessments conducted by the school psychologist, school nurse, and special education teacher.

This is, of course, much longer than the prior examples but still contains very little information unique to a particular child. Although we appreciate the effort, other than describing the special education evaluation process, the only unique data are given in the listing of possible impairments. Unfortunately, the statement provides no information about the nature of these impairments and does little to help us understand why the school team is evaluating this specific child.

Another problem with the previous referral statements is that they refer to constructs (e.g., *social/emotional behavior, attention, cognitive processes*, and *difficulties in academic progress*) that do not have a commonly shared definition. Not only will readers such as parents and teachers not understand them, but also they do not have a commonly accepted meaning among psychologists. This, unfortunately, means that no one who reads these reports will have anything more than a vague idea of what concerns led to the referral.

The Reason for Referral section of the report should communicate the purpose of the evaluation and identify the areas of concern. In addition, to strengthen the legal defensibility of the evaluation, it should identify what disabilities are in question. In order to accomplish this purpose, the Reason for Referral section should: (a) concisely describe the background or recent history of the problem; (b) describe the concerns, behaviors, or symptoms that led to the referral; (c) identify what areas or domains are to be assessed; and (d) communicate what disabilities are suspected. As much as possible, this section of the report should describe the concerns in behavioral terms. It can also be useful to quote the persons making the referral, using their words to describe the problem (Ownby, 1997). This information should logically lead to explicit evaluation questions or hypotheses, which we will discuss in more detail in the next section.

One implication of this approach is that the Reason for Referral section will often be longer than is typical in most reports, perhaps two or three paragraphs. The good news is that many reports already contain this information and it is simply a matter of moving some of what is usually placed in a background section into the Reason for Referral section.

When written more comprehensively, the Reason for Referral section of the report helps document the legal mandate that we assess in all areas of suspected disability and areas of need. In addition, it focuses the evaluation and makes it more individualized for a particular child. As we discussed in Chapters 2 and 3, this often requires that we spend time up front gathering information and exploring the problem with parents and teachers. Ahead we offer some examples and a discussion about their structure.

Examples: Reasons for Referral

Michael is a third-grade student at Neighborhood Elementary School. The school psychologist, speech-and-language therapist, and resource specialist teacher evaluated him earlier this school year because of concerns about his progress in reading as well as being off-task, talking out in class, being out of his seat without permission, and what his teacher described as "negative attention-seeking behavior." Michael's mother, Mrs. Smith, says that she has been concerned about his academic progress and behaviors in the classroom since he entered second grade last year. Despite these problems, the assessment team at Neighborhood concluded that Michael did not have a learning disability or an attention-deficit/hyperactivity disorder and did not require special education services. Mrs. Smith disputed this conclusion and requested further assessment because of her concerns about Michael's lack of friends and "odd" behaviors on the playground, such as playing alone or restlessly moving from one activity to another. On DATE, an assessment plan was signed for further evaluation of Michael's academic skills, intellectual development, speech and language skills, psychomotor development, self-help, and social-emotional development. Specifically, Mrs. Smith asked the team to address the possibility that Michael may have autism or an emotional disturbance.

Kris's school records show that she earned good grades up until ninth grade when she failed three classes. This semester she is failing Language Arts and Algebra. Kris has missed 20 days of school this semester and her teachers in Language Arts and Algebra report she only completes about 50% of her class and home-work. Kris's parents describe her as depressed and report five suicide attempts since March of last school year. Two of these resulted in hospitalizations. Both her parents and school personnel are concerned about her depression and her cur-rent ability to cope with the demands of high school. This evaluation will focus on Kris's social and emotional functioning and address the possibility that Kris has an emotional disturbance and needs special education assistance to make adequate progress toward high school graduation.

James is a fourth-grade student whom the Student Success Team and his mother referred for an evaluation because of concerns regarding his academic progress in reading and written language. During the last semester of this school year, James received interventions from the reading specialist for 90 minutes a week. The goal of these interventions was to increase his reading fluency and writing skills. Despite these interventions, his progress in reading and writing has been limited and he is at risk for not meeting the standards for promotion to fifth grade. The focus of this evaluation is to determine if James has a learning disability and what supports might help him to meet grade-level academic standards.

Sandy is a ninth-grade student who was referred for assessment by her mother, Ms. Hernandez, because of concerns about her academic progress. Specifically, Ms. Hernandez reports that Sandy is struggling with mathematics and complains that the work is too difficult for her. Although Ms. Hernandez's main concern is with Sandy's performance in mathematics, she is also doing poorly in several classes,

(continued)

> *(continued)*
>
> *despite receiving additional academic support since enrolling at Local Charter High School. For example, she has worked with the English-language support specialist and attended after-school tutoring for the last semester. Because of this, a psychoeducational assessment is being conducted in order to determine what types of supports or services Sandy requires in order to make adequate progress toward state and district academic standards. The eligibility addressed in this evaluation is Specific Learning Disability.*

Each of the previous paragraphs communicates information about the recent history of the problem. For example, we know that Michael's mother has been concerned about his academic progress and behavior for at least a year. We know that he was evaluated because of a suspected learning disability and ADHD and that the team did not find him eligible for special education services. We also know that Mrs. Smith is not content with that conclusion and wants the team to look into autism and emotional disturbance. Lastly, we know that the evaluation will cover a variety of domains, including academic skills, intellectual development, speech and language skills, psychomotor development, self-help, and social-emotional development.

We also know something about the symptoms or behaviors that have led to the referral for an evaluation. For Michael, we know that his mother believes he is not doing well in reading and that she and his teacher have been concerned about his being off-task, being out of his seat without permission, and "negative attention-seeking behavior." For Kris, we know she is failing classes, misses classes frequently, and only completes about half of her work. We also know that her parents are concerned about depression and that she has attempted suicide five times. In each case, we also know what disabilities are *suspected*, moving us closer to meeting our legal obligation to assess in all areas of suspected disability and need.

Clearly, there are still questions. We do not really know why Michael's mother has requested that the team focus on autism or emotional disturbance (other than that LD and ADHD were ruled out by the team first time around). There is obviously more to Kris's story of five suicide attempts and how the suspected depression is manifesting other than poor attendance and work completion. Yet, when compared with the examples at the beginning of this section, these do a much better job of giving the reader the context and rationale for the referral.

We have found that there is a balance in writing the reasons for evaluation between too little and too much. Too little does not communicate sufficient information for the reader to understand what concerns led to the evaluation and what the hypotheses are about the cause of these problems (see the examples at the beginning of this section). Too much detail makes the Reason for Referral section cumbersome to read. The goal is to provide a brief, though specific, introduction to what follows, which will of course have much more detail.

The referral concerns lead to the referral, or evaluation questions. The evaluation questions should follow logically from the description of the concerns contained in the narrative of the Reason for Referral section. Together with the information in the Reason for Referral section, they provide a focus and guide for the evaluation.

TRY IT!

WRITE A REASON FOR REFERRAL

Using information from one of your reports, write a Reason for Referral that communicates the following:

1. Brief history of the problem
2. A description of the behaviors or symptoms related to the problems
3. The areas of need and the suspected disabilities

Make sure that the information is unique to this child and his or her situation rather than generic.

HOW DO I DEVELOP WELL-FORMED EVALUATION QUESTIONS?

The information discussed in the Reason for Referral section should lead to explicit evaluation questions. In Batsche's Referral-Based Consultative Assessment/Report Writing Model, after reviewing existing information about a student, the next step is to collaboratively develop the referral questions (1983). Like Batsche's model, there should be a logical connection between the narrative of the Reason for Referral section and the evaluation questions that follow. Moreover, there should be logical connections between each aspect of the evaluation, including the reasons for the evaluation, the evaluation questions, the procedures chosen to conduct the evaluation, the results, and the recommendations that follow from the evaluation. This means that a reader should see the logical connection and flow between each stage of the evaluation.

We represent this in Figure 4.1 as a continuous cycle that starts from a discussion of concerns and ends with the identification of strengths and needs. The cycle can of course start

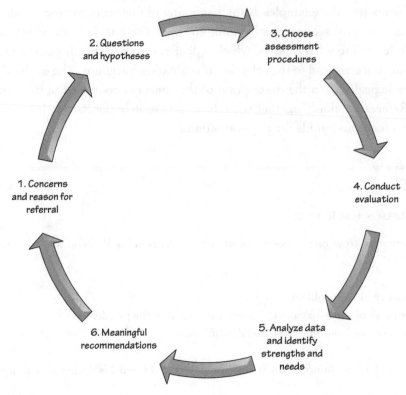

Figure 4.1   Evaluation Cycle

over, if there are new concerns or if the recommendations made do not adequately meet the identified needs. Like a good story plot, making our logic transparent goes a long way toward making reports more accessible and engaging to readers.

There is a legal framework for the types of questions that the evaluation must answer. Section 300.304 of IDEA notes the questions that an evaluation must answer:

In conducting the evaluation, the public agency must:

1. Use a variety of assessment tools and strategies to gather relevant functional, developmental, and academic information about the child, including information provided by the parent that may assist in determining—
    i.   Whether the child is a child with a disability under Sec. 300.8; and
    ii.   The content of the child's IEP, including information related to enabling the child to be involved in and progress in the general education curriculum [emphasis added]. (IDEA, 2004)

We interpret (i) and (ii) as framing two types of questions for all evaluations: (1) disability or diagnostic questions, and (2) recommendations or "What do we need to do differently?" questions. Given that we are also responsible to assess in all areas of need related to the disability, and the psychoeducational evaluation is the foundation for the IEP, we add a third type of question, (3) current levels of functioning questions. In our reports we typically put the present-levels questions first, the diagnostic questions(s) second, and the "What do we need to do differently?" question last. In the following sections we discuss each of these in turn.

HOW DO I WRITE PRESENT LEVELS OF FUNCTIONING QUESTIONS?

Present-levels questions connect to the mandate to assess in all areas of need, whether or not they relate directly to the disabilities in question. They can, of course, vary depending on the child in question and the concerns raised by teachers or parents, but they often correspond to the areas listed on a typical assessment plan, for example, academic skills (reading, written language, and math), cognitive functioning, social emotional functioning, and so on. Samples of present-levels questions that correspond to the cases of Michael and Kris could include:

1. ***What are Michael's current levels of academic, cognitive, psychomotor, and social and emotional development?***
2. ***What are Kris's current levels of academic, cognitive, and social and emotional development?***

These examples of present-levels questions combine different areas of concern into one question. Although this may be appropriate in some situations, it can often be clearer to state each of these as a separate question. For example, Kris's questions could be rewritten as three separate questions:

1. ***What is Kris's level of academic development?***
2. ***What is Kris's level of cognitive development?***
3. ***What is Kris's level of social and emotional development?***

Returning to the section of IDEA that discusses evaluations, certain areas are specifically mentioned in the law:

(4) The child is assessed in *all* areas related to the suspected disability, including, if appropriate, health, vision, hearing, social and emotional status, general intelligence, academic performance, communicative status, and motor abilities [emphasis added]. (IDEA, 2004)

Given that school psychologists work in education, the issue of academic performance is always relevant in one way or another. For some children, the issue will be one of academic skill development, and for others, like Kris, who appear to have adequate skills, the more important issue will be one of classroom performance and the influence of motivation or the presence of behaviors that interfere with studying, completing work, or following classroom routines, such as inattention and impulsivity.

As we have discussed in Chapter 3, we also advocate for incorporating strengths into evaluations and reports. Returning to the present-level question above, they could be phrased to guide the evaluation to account for strengths and needs rather than just a level of functioning. For example, Kris's present-level question, "What are Kris's current levels of academic, cognitive, and social and emotional development?" would become "What are Kris's academic, cognitive, and social and emotional strengths and needs?" If we separated them into three different questions, they would be:

1. *What are Kris's academic strengths and needs?*
2. *What are Kris's cognitive strengths and needs?*
3. *What are Kris's social emotional strengths and needs?*

Some school districts require that *every* child who is referred for an evaluation be assessed in certain areas. For example, every student is given a standardized test of intelligence or achievement, no matter the concerns raised by those who made the referral. This seems unnecessary, inefficient, and even intrusive. If there is good evidence from a child's history that his academic skills are adequate (e.g., grades, work samples, district academic benchmarks, state testing, etc.), then it seems sufficient to use these data, usually gathered through reviews of records and interviews, to document the student's present levels. Remember, we need to collect relevant data to help the IEP team write goals and create interventions. In this case, through our review of records and interviews we collected the relevant data needed and there is no reason to give a standardized achievement test. This allows the busy school psychologist to spend her or his limited time focusing on assessment concerns that are a higher priority instead of giving unwarranted standardized batteries.

District mandates that require the administration of a certain kind of standardized assessment seem to arise from a perspective that treats data from standardized tests as more legally defensible. We know of no evidence that suggests this is true. If called to testify regarding an evaluation, the standards by which that testimony would be judged would be similar to those used to judge expert witnesses and their testimony. If we examine how courts treat this issue, there is clearly room for judgments based on interpretation of the facts that draws upon professional knowledge and experience (Fed. R. Evid. 702 advisory committee's note, 2000 amendments). Legally, psychologists are required to support their opinions, whether it involves use of a standardized test or professional judgment based on other kinds of assessment data.

TRY IT!

IDENTIFY WHICH DOMAINS OF CONCERN NEED TO BE EVALUATED

1. Reread one of your recent reports. Based on what you knew before the evaluation, what areas do you need to assess?
2. For each of these areas of need, write a question that would guide the evaluation.

How Do I Write Diagnostic or Disability Questions?

Simply put, legally all evaluations must determine whether a child has a disability and, if so, what kind. As we discussed in Chapters 2 and 3, it is good practice to identify what disabilities are in question up front, as part of the pre-assessment process. This is not only good practice but helpful in documenting your efforts to meet the legal mandate to assess in all areas of suspected disability. This is one of the problems with the poorly written referral examples on page 66. Although it identifies areas of potential impairment, it does not identify the suspected disabilities. We, as experienced professionals, could read between the lines and guess Other Health Impaired (because of possible ADHD implied by problems with attention) or Emotional Disturbance (implied by impairments of social/emotional functioning), but given the lack of other information, this is dangerously vague and not useful for those reading the report. We believe that it is much better to state explicitly the suspected disabilities in the questions that guide the evaluation.

The disability questions themselves are straightforward. There are 13 disabilities listed in IDEA (see Table 4.1). In most cases, you will quickly eliminate many of them because of your prior knowledge of the student's concerns (e.g., deaf-blind, orthopedic impairment, etc.). Choosing the remaining suspected disabilities will depend on the quality of information you have at the beginning stages of the assessment process and your ability to clarify the referring parties' concerns and formulate hypotheses.

We often use the assessment plan itself as a guide. As we go through each area listed on the plan (e.g., academic skills, cognitive ability, motor skills, etc.), we ask the parent and teacher about their perceptions of the student's strengths and weaknesses in each area. If something is not stated as an area of concern, we will ask questions that help us understand why this is not a concern. If something is stated as a concern (i.e., "Adrian just can't

Table 4.1   Disability Categories in IDEA 2004

Autism	Other health impairment
Deaf-blindness	Orthopedic impairment
Deafness	Specific learning disability
Emotional disturbance	Speech or language impairment
Hearing impairment	Traumatic brain injury
Intellectual disability	Visual impairment (including blindness)
Multiple disabilities	

seem to remember what I tell him to do"), we ask questions that help clarify what this looks like and what might be underlying this problem. For example, we would want to know if Adrian's difficulty with remembering instructions was related to attention, motivation, memory, or some combination of these factors. During this process, we will sometimes ask direct questions such as "Do you think Adrian has a learning disability?" or "Has anyone ever mentioned autism to you in talking about Adrian's difficulties?" This back-and-forth conversation inevitably narrows down our list of suspected disabilities and helps us identify what domains are of concern. Although not directly related to this topic, this early collaboration with parents and teachers also helps the IEP members feel like participants in the evaluation process, rather than uninvolved observers while we conduct our assessments.

Using Michael's sample Reason for Referral statement, we can reasonably develop evaluation questions that focus on identifying a short list of suspected disabilities. For example, *Does Michael have autism or an emotional disturbance, as defined by IDEA?* In Michael's case, the most important reason for these disabilities to be included is that his mother has requested that the evaluation focus on them. In other words, Michael's mother suspects them, so they automatically go on to the list of concerns we discussed in Chapter 2. There is some evidence that supports these hypotheses, such as lack of friendships and odd behavior on the playground, but from a conservative legal perspective, Mrs. Smith's concerns trump the school personnel's opinion about the strength of this evidence.

Does Kris have an emotional disturbance as defined by federal and state regulations? This question seems more straightforward. Kris earned good grades before high school, which does not give strong support to a learning disability. The concerns focus on depression, suicide attempts, poor school attendance, and poor work completion. Given this, it seems logical that an emotional disturbance would be the strongest hypothesis for an educational disability.

TRY IT!

IDENTIFY THE SUSPECTED DISABILITIES

1. Reread one of your recent reports. Based on what you knew before the evaluation, what disabilities do you suspect?
2. For each of these suspected disabilities, write a question that would guide the evaluation.

HOW DO I WRITE SOLUTION-BASED, OR "WHAT DO WE DO ABOUT THIS" QUESTIONS?

The last type of question is the "What do we do about this?" question. It is in our response to this question that we make the recommendations that flow from our identification of the child's strengths and needs. If needed, this is also where we make recommendations about the content of a child's individualized education program. We often phrase this as two questions. One question focuses on what might be necessary for the child to make adequate progress as judged by academic standards. The second asks if special education is necessary in order to accomplish this. Examples of these questions for both an initial evaluation and a reevaluation follow.

Examples: "What Do We Do About This?" — Initial Referral Questions

1. *What supports are necessary to help Michael make adequate progress toward state and district academic standards? Does he need special education services in order to meet these expectations?*
2. *What changes to James's current educational program are needed for him to make adequate progress toward state and district academic standards?*
3. *What accommodations or interventions are necessary to help Kris better manage her symptoms of depression and anxiety at school?*

Examples: "What Do We Do About This?" — Triennial or Three-Year Reevaluation Questions

1. *What, if any, additions or changes to Nolan's special education and related services are needed to help him to meet his annual goals and to participate, as appropriate, in the general education curriculum?*

(continued)

(continued)

2. *What additional interventions or services are needed for Hanh to continue to make adequate progress toward her goals in reading and written language?*
3. *What accommodations or interventions would assist Sean to make adequate progress toward high school graduation?*
4. *Is Lily's placement in a special day class meeting her educational needs?*

These types of questions put the issue of "What do you do about this?" and our recommendations front and center in our reports. Once evaluation questions are developed, the school psychologist determines what evaluation tools to use and what data to collect to answer these questions. It is beyond the scope of this book to delve into assessment practices and tools for each area of suspected disability; however, we hope you keep in mind the legal and best practice assessment points we have highlighted:

- The evaluation should be comprehensive.
- The evaluator should use a variety of assessment tools or approaches that gather functional and relevant data.
- The evaluation should be fair.
- The evaluator should be competent.
- The procedures used should be valid and reliable.

In the following sections, we discuss how to use evaluation questions as the structure for your reports. We also discuss how to write background information, assessment themes, and good recommendations.

TRY IT!

PULLING IT ALL TOGETHER TO WRITE EVALUATION QUESTIONS

Using information from one of your reports, write at least three questions that would guide your evaluation:

1. Present-levels question (domains or areas of need that need to be evaluated)
2. Disability question (suspected disabilities)
3. "What do we do about it?" question (needed accommodations and interventions)

THE BACKGROUND INFORMATION PROVIDES DEVELOPMENTAL AND EDUCATIONAL PERSPECTIVE TO YOUR REPORT

The background information in a report has two important purposes. The first is to provide sufficient information about children to situate them in a developmental, social, and educational context. To return to our analogy of report as a story, it is important to know enough about the protagonist of a story in order to understand the implications of the plot. In the same way, it is important that we have enough basic information (e.g., gender, age, grade, family composition, etc.), in order to understand both the concerns and the results of the evaluation.

The second purpose of the background information is to identify social, health, or developmental factors that might play a role in explaining the concerns raised by consumers. Examples might include a previously unidentified hearing problem or a history of poor attendance and limited access to instruction. These factors can play a role in decision making by either their presence or their absence. The presence of symptoms early in development can play a direct role in diagnosing such disabilities as an intellectual disability, autism, or attention-deficit/hyperactivity disorder (ADHD). The absence of certain background variables can also play a role in deciding that a lack of academic progress is best explained by a lack of instruction or a health condition rather than a learning disability or that a child's symptoms of hyperactivity are caused by ADHD rather than lack of sleep or medication taken for an illness. The background information can be structured in two ways. One is to give it the heading of *Background Information* as would be typical in most report structures. The second is to present it as a question, similar to the questions we have discussed. An example of how the Background section can be framed as a question is:

How does Anthony's developmental, health, and educational history affect his academic achievement?

Either way, it is important to begin this section with an explanation of the source of the information we report. As with other aspects of the evaluation, this makes clear the sources of our information and any potential limitations of the data we have gathered.

Examples: Providing Sources of Background Information

> *Background information about Diego was obtained from a review of his school records and Mrs. Brown's responses to questions on the Behavioral Assessment for Children–3 Structured Developmental History (BASC SDH).*
>
> ~
>
> (*continued*)

(continued)

Kim's background information was gathered from the Multidisciplinary Assessment Team Report written in February of DATE, a Structured Developmental History completed by Mrs. Brady, and an interview with Mr. and Mrs. Brady on DATE.

The background information below was gathered from a school district health and developmental history form completed by Mrs. Johnson, a Multidisciplinary Team Report written in February of DATE, Randy's school records, an interview with Randy, and a phone interview with Mrs. Johnson.

Following this introduction, we must make important decisions about what to include or not include in this section. One of the common challenges we face is sorting through the large amount of background information gathered during an evaluation and determining what information is important to highlight. This decision has both ethical and practical implications.

First, it is important to understand the scope of our evaluation. This helps us answer the question, "Is this relevant?" We have advocated for clearly stating the reasons for the evaluation and for developing questions that will guide the evaluation. This helps us understand the scope or purpose of the evaluation before we start, but also helps us communicate that purpose to the readers. Communicating the purpose of the evaluation clearly is not only an important aspect of informed consent and developing a collaborative relationship with consumers, but it can also help us decide what is relevant to include in a report. If the information we have gathered does not assist us in answering the evaluation questions we have posed, it is probably not pertinent and should not be included.

Second, the first goal of most ethical codes is typically *beneficence*, or the duty to do no harm. Given this, in addition to asking if the information helps us tell the story of a child accurately or if it helps us answer one of the evaluation questions, it is important to ask also if the information will do harm or break confidentiality in unnecessary ways (Michaels, 2006).

There is, of course, a tension in answering these two questions. Revealing a mother's drug use during pregnancy may be helpful in understanding a child's symptoms of hyperactivity but may also embarrass or deepen a sense of guilt or shame she has about the experience. In the spirit of a collaborative relationship, we will often either ask if it is okay to put a sensitive piece of information in a report or, if we have strong feelings that it is necessary, will at least frontload the parent (or child) that the information will be included and what our rationale is.

The Background Information Provides Developmental and Educational Perspective

There are many ways to sequence or structure the information in the Background section but we often start by situating the child in a family. With bilingual youth, this is also where we will discuss language usage.

Examples: Situating the Child in a Family

Peter is an only child who lives at home with his mother and stepfather. Mrs. Lopez separated from Peter's biological father when he was about nine months old. When interviewed, Peter said he does not see his biological father and described him as "out of the picture." Peter has three half-siblings but he has little contact with them. Mrs. Lopez and Peter's stepfather have been together for about 12 years.

Kendra lives at home with her father and her paternal grandmother. Mrs. and Mr. Endo have been divorced since Kendra was about 6 months old. According to her father, Kendra sees her mother weekly for an hour or less.

Antonio lives at home with his parents, his twin brother, a 9-year-old sister, and a 2-year-old brother. Antonio's mother is from Guatemala and Antonio's family lived in Guatemala off and on until he was about 3 years old. Mrs. Gonzales reports that she has always spoken English to Antonio and he does not speak Spanish.

Note that both Peter and Kendra live in families where there has been a divorce. This is a good example of potentially sensitive information. Our decision in these cases is that this is important basic information for understanding these families and potential sources of social support or stress. We would be cautious beyond this basic information. For example, it is probably not worth mentioning that Peter's mother had mentioned she was "disgusted" by her ex-husband's "fooling around and wasting money" behavior. This information is likely not pertinent to the referral questions and has at least some potential for harm. We understand that there might be situations where the tension between separated parents or other family issues may play an important role in explaining a child's problems. As we mentioned earlier, we think it is best practice to discuss this with the parent beforehand. We are also cautious about interpreting or putting our own spin on this kind of information and will often use the informants' own words to describe the situation. For example, we might say, "Mrs. Lopez describes her relationship with Peter's father as 'difficult' and says the separation has been 'very difficult on both me and Peter.'"

We typically follow this section with information about the birth, early development, and health. This is the part of the Background section where we also describe the child's current health status, including any medical concerns and treatment, as well as current vision and hearing. We encourage writers of reports to phrase information positively. In other words, rather than saying, "Mike did not have any problems at birth and his mother says he did not experience any developmental delays," we prefer to say, "Mike and his mother were healthy at his birth. His mother reports that he met his early developmental milestones within typical time frames." The goal here is not to gloss over negative experiences or challenges, but whenever possible, describe the presence of something rather than the absence of something. For example, someone is "healthy" rather than "does not have any health problems." This is not only easier to understand for the average consumer but also avoids the off-putting use of unnecessarily negative language in our reports. Some examples of this section include the following.

Examples: Using Positive Language

Steve and Mrs. O'Connell were healthy during the pregnancy and birth. Mrs. O'Connell reports that he had a heart murmur at birth but this resolved itself without treatment by the time he was one year old. Steve had four ear infections, though was healthy as a young child. Steve met all early developmental milestones; however, when he started school at the age of 6, he had difficulties with over-activity, paying attention to classroom work, and immature social skills. He is currently healthy and has normal vision and hearing.

Mrs. Johnson describes herself as having had "emotional problems" during her pregnancy with Jake. She also smoked during the pregnancy but, despite this, Jake and his mother were healthy at his birth. Mrs. Johnson describes Jake as a "happy baby" and says that he met his early developmental milestones within typical time limits. He currently uses an inhaler to treat seasonal asthma as needed.

Mrs. Cortez reports that Juan was born with a congenital heart disease, causing one of his chambers to atrophy. He had a shunt inserted at 3 months and underwent

---

> *open-heart surgery at 10 and 18 months. At 18 months of age, he had a pacemaker inserted, which was replaced with a new device when he was 3 years old. Juan took Lasix from 3 months of age until he was 2 years old. He does not currently take any medications and there are no restrictions on his physical activity. His parents describe him as healthy and school records indicate normal vision and hearing. Despite the heart disease, Juan's parents report that he met his early developmental milestones within typical time limits and, other than the heart problems, he was healthy as a young child.*

After providing information about birth, early development, and health, we will also discuss any prior community-based evaluations and treatment. If the child was evaluated by a school district, we usually incorporate these data into the Education History section that follows.

Examples: Medical or Treatment History

> *In February of DATE, Brady Adams, PhD, evaluated Connie following a referral from her mother. In a report, dated DATE, Dr. Adams states that Connie was referred for an assessment because of "her lack of attention and concentration (difficulty organizing tasks and forgetfulness), hyperactive behavior (fidgeting and talking excessively), and because of excessive anxiety." In the summary of his report, Dr. Adams described Connie as having above-average intellectual functioning based on her performance on the Wechsler Intelligence Scale for Children. He also described her academic skills as "appropriate" although she was slightly below grade level in spelling per her scores on the Wide Range Achievement Test. He concludes by stating that the "best" diagnosis for Connie at the time was generalized anxiety disorder. Although Dr. Adams noted that Connie had a prior diagnosis of attention-deficit/hyperactivity disorder, combined type (ADHD), he states that because her problems with inattention and hyperactivity did not seem to occur at school, her problems were better accounted for by anxiety than by ADHD.*
>
> ---
>
> *Although her early development seemed typical, Mr. and Mrs. Guthrie sought medical treatment for Mia beginning at age 5 because of problems at school with*
>
> *(continued)*

(continued)

over-activity, paying attention to classroom work, and immature social skills. Initially, Mia was diagnosed with attention-deficit/hyperactivity disorder (ADHD) and treated with stimulant medication. Over time, Mia's treating psychiatrists have also suggested possible diagnoses of bipolar disorder and obsessive-compulsive disorder (OCD) because of tantrums, mood swings, and extreme attachment to objects that Mr. and Mrs. Guthrie call her "security blankets." Because of these problems, Mia was treated with Abilify (aripiprazole), a medication used to treat symptoms of aggression, mood swings, and temper tantrums. Mia currently takes Adderall, a stimulant medication used to treat ADHD, and Abilify. Dr. Randy Kennedy is Mia's current psychiatrist. He sees Mia monthly to review her response to her medication.

In fourth grade, Albert saw Dr. Pearcy, a psychologist in private practice. In a letter dated DATE, Dr. Pearcy writes that he had seen Albert for "counseling and consultation." He goes on to state that Albert's mind wanders and he has difficulty focusing and attending for "more than a minimal level of time." Dr. Pearcy also describes Albert as having difficulty with organization and planning and says he is "not hyper in any way but clearly inattentive." In his letter, Dr. Pearcy recommends further evaluation by the school psychologist and requests that Albert's workload be reduced as an accommodation to his difficulties with attention and "executive functions."

Following the information about birth, early development, and health, we would typically discuss the child's educational history. This can vary considerably depending on a child's educational experiences. The following are examples of an initial referral with a complex history, an initial evaluation with a less complex history, and a special education reevaluation.

Examples: Educational History

Max is in the fifth grade at Ideal Elementary School. Max's school records are incomplete because he has changed school many times. Max attended Kindergarten through the second trimester of second grade at Super Elementary School in Quality Unified School District. Max had poor attendance in Kindergarten and his initial year in first grade. He repeated first grade, though his attendance remained poor. Max was provided interventions while enrolled at Super Elementary, including small-group instruction, summer school, and at-risk Resource Specialist Program (RSP) services. Max's school records did not contain information about how well these interventions worked.

Max transferred to Major Elementary in Another Unified School District to complete second grade. He was involved in a summer reading clinic then returned to Major for third grade. During the third grade, the Student Study Team discussed Max's academic progress, and, according to his mother, the team recommended an assessment for special education services. She remembers that the evaluation concluded that Max had "perceptual problems" but the team did not think he needed special education services. The report was not available to review for this evaluation.

Max began attending school within the Current Unified School District (CUSD) on DATE. He attended fourth grade at Hope School, a school exclusively for students who are homeless. He transferred to Ideal Elementary School on DATE as a fifth grader. Since enrolling at Ideal, Max has had good attendance.

According to his mother, Heng attended full-day preschool two or three days a week starting when he was 3 years old. He started Kindergarten at Kelly Elementary when he was 5 years old. At the end of Kindergarten, the school discussed retention with Mrs. Le because Heng had made limited progress in early reading skills and there were concerns that he was not ready for first grade. Despite these concerns, Heng was promoted to first grade. He is currently in a second-grade class but goes to an extra reading group twice a week for 30 minutes in a first-grade classroom.

Claudia has received special education services since Kindergarten. At different times since Kindergarten, she has been classified as a student with a developmental

(continued)

> *(continued)*
>
> *delay, a speech and language impairment, or a learning disability; however, her current eligibility is Specific Learning Disability (SLD). Claudia received special education services in a special day class from first through eighth grade. She repeated fifth grade because her mother did not believe that Claudia was mature enough for middle school and requested retention. Claudia is currently in ninth grade at Local City High School in a combination of general education classes, general education classes with push-in special education support, and special education classes.*

Some authors include information about a child's hobbies, friendships, relationships with parents, and so on in the Background section. For the most part, we have found that this information is better placed in the Evaluation Results section as part of our response to the evaluation questions. For many of the children we evaluate, their social and emotional functioning is a concern. Given this, information about these topics, even if it is historical, is usually important in answering an evaluation question regarding their emotional status and ability to get along well with peers and adults. In addition, in the next section we will further discuss how developing and answering specific evaluation questions pushes us to integrate different sources and kinds of data and look past the kinds of categories found in test-based and domain-based report structures.

ASSESSMENT DATA FROM MULTIPLE SOURCES IS INTEGRATED INTO THEMES

If you were writing a report using the approach we advocate, you would so far have: (a) a Reason for Referral section that explains the rationale and purpose of the evaluation; (b) a short list of evaluation questions; and (c) a Background section that provides the developmental, health, social, and educational context for the referral. What would typically follow this in a more traditional report would be an Evaluation Results section that would perhaps be divided into subheadings based on the instruments you used (a test-based format) or domains of functioning (a domain-based report). Instead, we recommend that you use the evaluation questions as the basic structure for your Evaluation Results section. As we mentioned at the beginning of this chapter, we recommend you put the present-levels questions first, the disability question second, and the "What do we need to do differently?" question last.

Example: Referral-Based Report Structure

For Kris, the headings for your report might be:

1. Reason for referral
2. Evaluation questions
3. Background
4. Evaluation results
   a. What are Kris's academic strengths and needs?
   b. What are Kris's cognitive strengths and needs?
   c. What is Kris's level of social emotional development?
   d. Does Kris have an emotional disturbance as defined by federal and state regulations?
   e. What supports are necessary to help Kris make adequate progress toward state and district academic standards? Does she need special education services in order to meet these expectations?

With this model, you first pose and then answer the questions. Questions 4a–e become the subheadings for your Evaluation Results section. In many reports, interpretation and integration of data is left to the Conclusion or Summary section. Our reports do not contain a summary or conclusion because the interpretation and integration of assessment data is ongoing and explicit in how we answer the evaluation questions. We agree with Batsche (1983) that integration of assessment data should occur throughout the report and believe this structure lends itself to the greatest integration of data.

We want to be clear about the implications of this. For example, we do not have an "observations" section or an "interview" section but rather all information is integrated throughout the report. The response to an evaluation question may draw upon history, interview data, observations, or test results. Figure 4.2 represents how we conceptualize this.

This approach is challenging for us as authors because it forces us to think through all of the data we have gathered for the information that helps us answer each of the evaluation questions. This moves us in the direction of integrating different types of data to answer the question, a clear legal as well as best practice mandate. For example, in question 4a it would be common for us to discuss teacher reports, state testing, district benchmarks, and standardized academic test batteries. In the answer to the second question, 4b, we might include developmental information, teacher and parent reports, and the results of a standardized assessment of cognitive skills.

Within each section of the evaluation results, we will often use theme statements as another organizing tool. A theme statement is a concise (from one to three sentences) summary of the

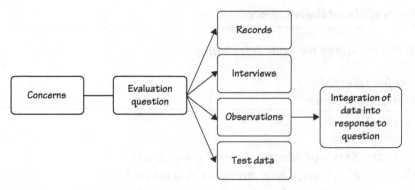

Figure 4.2   Integration of Information in Response to Evaluation Question

information that follows. One way to think about this is if we lifted the questions and themes statements from a report, we would essentially have an outline of our evaluation. Another way to understand the themes is that they are the answers to our evaluation questions. They are our major findings or conclusions, which, instead of being placed in a summary or conclusion, are integrated throughout the report as responses to the evaluation questions. In addition to being concise, theme statements should be written in straightforward language without reference to technical data. We typically highlight theme statements by using bold or italic type or placing them in text boxes in our reports. We will also usually place a statement at the beginning of the Evaluation Results section before our findings or responses to the evaluation questions, to explain the question-based format to the reader. An example of this is:

The assessment questions addressed within this report are listed as headings below. After each question, the answer is provided in italics. The information and data used to answer the questions are also provided in the narrative following each question. Specific scores on standardized assessments are included on the last page of the report.

We provide sample theme statements taken from our reports in what follows. Some are in response to present-levels questions and some in response to disability questions.

Examples: Sample Theme Statements

Although Kris has average cognitive ability and academic skills, she failed three classes last year and is failing two classes this semester. She has completed 50 of 180 credits required for high school graduation with a 2.0 GPA.

Henry has average basic academic skills for his grade but he appears to have difficulty when he has to apply these skills to reading comprehension, oral math, or written expression. He seems to be making good progress toward the academic goals on his IEP and is reported to work best one-on-one or in small groups.

⟞⟝

Eva's pre-academic achievement was assessed through review of records, observations, teacher reports, interviews, and classroom work samples. Overall, Eva has made progress toward many academic preschool standards, though her limited language skills and behaviors affect her ability to engage meaningfully in classroom activities.

⟞⟝

Jacob appears to have average academic skills and he has passed the high school exit exam. He is currently earning A's and B's in academic classes and is on track to graduate from high school at the end of the next school year.

⟞⟝

Melanie appears to be academically underachieving relative to her age and ability, especially in reading and written expression. Her verbal abilities are strong as well as her ability to hear, identify, and work with individual sounds but significant limitations in short-term memory and the ability to focus on a task and work quickly are impacting her reading decoding and fluency skills.

What follows each theme statement is a narrative that supports the theme by providing information integrated from various sources. This is a key point; rather than categorize information by domains or by the instrument used, it is organized so it responds to the evaluation questions posed. To return to our metaphor of report as story, the goal is to present a coherent plot that the reader can follow, using the questions as the basic structure. As to how much information is adequate to support a theme, we again suggest using Merrell's *Rule of Two* and RIOT as guides (Leung, 1993; Levitt & Merrell, 2009). Two examples of what the combination of question, theme statement, and supporting data might look like follow. To see more examples, refer to Appendix II at the end of the book.

Examples: Pulling It All Together—Question, Theme (Answer), and Data

---

1. What are Kris's cognitive and academic strengths and needs?

Although Kris has average cognitive ability and academic skills, she failed three classes last year and is failing two classes this semester. She has completed 50 of 180 credits required for high school graduation with a 2.0 GPA.

As of January of DATE, Kris had completed 50 of the 180 credits needed for high school graduation with a cumulative grade point average of 2.0. She failed three classes her ninth grade year, which leaves her 15 credits behind what is typical after completing ninth grade. Kris has not yet taken the High School Exit Exam.

At the end of the second quarter of the fall semester, Kris had A's in Choir and Athletics. She had C's in World History and Language Arts and F's in Algebra and Biology. Both low test scores and missing or incomplete assignments are noted in the teacher comments on her report card for the classes she is failing. In Choir, the teacher noted she was a "pleasure to have in class."

In February of DATE, Kris was given both the Woodcock Johnson IV Tests of Achievement (WJ IV ACH) and the Woodcock Johnson IV Tests of Cognitive Ability (WJ COG). On the WJ COG, Kris's general intellectual ability was average. She had significant strengths in auditory processing and short-term memory, including working memory. Academically, Kris's performance on the WJ ACH in reading, written language, and math were all in the average range.

---

2. How does Drew's developmental and educational history affect his current academic achievement?

Drew has a history of significant language delays. He was evaluated by Local Regional Center at 2 years, 8 months of age, and then referred to Local School District for an evaluation for special education. Drew has received special education services under the eligibility of Speech and Language Impairment since his initial evaluation in January of DATE. He initially received services through placement in a moderate-to-severe special day class, though his placement for Kindergarten was changed to a mild-moderate special day class. Drew has transitioned well to his new school and successfully participates in a general education classroom for 90 minutes a day.

Drew's background history was gathered through a review of his school cumulative records and an interview with his mother. Because of concerns with his language development, Drew was evaluated through Local Regional Center (LRC) in September of DATE. According to their evaluation, Drew's cognitive, physical, and social development were all typical for his age. At the same time, he was distractible, inattentive, and had difficulty with transitions. He also demonstrated significant delays in language development. LRC referred Drew to Local School District (LSD) for a special education evaluation in January of DATE. An Individualized Education Plan (IEP) meeting was held on DATE. According to the psychoeducational evaluation, Drew's nonverbal cognitive development was in the low-average-to-average range, though his short attention span negatively affected his performance on the tests used in the evaluation. His gross and fine-motor skills appear to be typical. His social skills were somewhat delayed and his adaptive skills were significantly delayed. Based on speech and language evaluation in both Spanish and English, Drew's expressive language, receptive language, and articulation were significantly delayed.

Drew qualified for special education services as a child with a speech and language impairment (SLI) because of significant delays in expressive language, receptive language, and articulation. Goals were written in listening and speaking and self-regulation. Drew was placed in a moderate-to-severe special day class (MS SDC) preschool program with 90 weekly minutes of speech and language services. He began attending First Elementary School in September of DATE.

Drew's first annual IEP meeting was held on DATE. He had met all five of his IEP goals. Drew continued in the MS SDC preschool program; however, his SL services were changed to 15 minutes of monthly collaboration. A second annual IEP was held on DATE. Drew had again met all of his IEP goals. An addendum meeting was held on DATE at the end of his final year of preschool. The team reviewed placement options for kindergarten and changed his placement to a mild-moderate special day class (MM SDC) at his home school, Second Elementary.

Note again the integration of different kinds of data in both examples. In a more traditional report, some of the information in Kris's example (e.g., grades, credits earned, etc.) might have been placed in a Background section or the Academic Achievement section. Here the question is answered by a combination of current information from school records and historical information from a prior evaluation. In Drew's example, information gathered through records review and a parent interview was combined to look at his history as a whole.

The number of themes is of course dependent on the question asked and the data gathered and there may be multiple themes throughout the answer of a question. A simple outline of what this might look like in a report would be:

1. Evaluation results
    a. What are Kris's academic strengths and needs?
        i. Theme 1
            1. Evaluation data
        ii. Theme 1
            1. Evaluation data

We have found this format to be especially helpful when talking to parents and teachers about the evaluation results. What we typically do is to start the conversation with a reminder of the concerns discussed in the early stages of the evaluation process and then move on to pose and answer each question in turn. The questions and theme statements provide a natural outline for discussing the results and the recommendations that follow.

To summarize, use theme statements as summary statements or subheadings in the narrative response to an evaluation question. The questions and theme statements are a way of structuring the Evaluation Results section so that it focuses explicitly on the questions raised by consumers. They are concise, written in straightforward, nontechnical language, and typically draw upon data across assessment methods or sources. Contrast this with a test-based or domain-based report, where the data are not usually integrated until the end of the report.

TRY IT!

WRITE THEME STATEMENTS

Using information from one of your reports, write one or more theme statements for one domain of functioning in the report. Remember to use straightforward language and to integrate information across assessment methods.

HOW DO I WRITE USEFUL RECOMMENDATIONS?

Recommendations are what consumers are waiting for. As we discussed in Chapter 3, consumers such as parents and teachers have a very practical view of evaluations, and although they may be impressed with diagnostic wizardry, they value most professional judgment about what needs to be done to improve things for their children and students. Despite this, recommendations are often ignored because they are too complex or vague, or do not appear directly related to consumers' concerns.

We have found some school psychologists reluctant to provide meaningful recommendations in their reports. Sometimes this seems to arise from the fear that schools districts will be legally obligated to provide whatever they put in writing. As we have argued, we believe this fear is overblown. So, if we were to state the first point of this section (in the spirit of the themes we discussed earlier), it would be to always provide meaningful recommendations.

In fact, we strongly believe that providing meaningful recommendations that respond to consumers' concerns is a very good way to avoid legal complications. Although there has been a great deal of discussion in our field for increased involvement by school psychologists in intervention and prevention, many school psychologists continue to function as special education gatekeepers. One of the many problems with this role is that too often parents will attend a meeting where evaluation results are discussed and, unless their child is eligible for special education, the team has little to offer in the way of recommendations for meaningful changes in the child's educational program. Recommendations are either nonexistent or so weak as to be of little use. If we view this from the perspective of a parent, the concerns that led to the referral remain but we have left them empty-handed. Many times, we have seen this frustration and dissatisfaction lead to requests for expensive independent educational evaluations and other time-consuming legal complications.

The process of crafting meaningful recommendations begins with the identification of the child's unique pattern of strengths and needs. Given the potential that these recommendations might end up as part of a child's Individualized Education Program (IEP) in one form or another, it is important that recommendations be individualized and respond to unique needs. The clear identification of unique need helps provide the rationale for the recommendation. As you can tell from this and other comments we have made, we strongly believe that generic information is seldom helpful to the reader or, more importantly, the child. This is especially true for generic recommendations that do seem to respond to a particular child's unique needs. These are both inadequate, legally, and ineffective (Yell, 1998). Even if a child does not need special education services and we are technically free of the mandate to develop an Individualized Education Plan, it is best practice to provide appropriate general education recommendations that respond to that child's unique needs. Given this, the second point of this section is to link recommendations to clearly identified needs.

Recommendations can range from general to very specific. Where one falls on this continuum can depend on many factors, including your knowledge and training, but also the context of where the recommendations are to be implemented (i.e., is it reasonable for this to be done in this classroom or this school, etc.). On one hand, it can be perceived as presumptuous to be overly detailed and prescriptive about what teachers do in their classrooms. On the other hand, we want to avoid writing recommendations that are so general or obvious that they are of no practical use or, worse, offend the reader by appearing too simplistic (e.g., "Provide multimodal presentation of information"). We have tended to be more specific when we are confident that what we are recommending can be accomplished in a particular setting. This assumes you know your school team and the persons who will implement the interventions. In cases where we know less or have less confidence, we are often more general and offer examples of the kinds of things that might meet the needs we have identified.

Once a child's needs have been clearly identified, it is helpful to have a way to conceptualize the kinds of recommendations you might make in a report. One way to understand types of recommendations is to see them in terms of (a) additional evaluation, (b) accommodations, (c) instructional or curriculum modifications, (d) specialized supports or services, and (e) referrals to a community agency or other resource (Lichtenberger et al., 2004; National Dissemination Center for Children with Disabilities [NICHCY], 2010). Figure 4.3 outlines this problem-solving process as it relates to recommendations. Once a student's unique strengths and needs are clarified, then meaningful recommendations can be written in the appropriate areas.

Recommendations for further evaluation are common when the results suggest that specialists not involved in the initial evaluation conduct additional evaluation. For example, this could arise when your assessment of a child's verbal abilities suggests the need for the

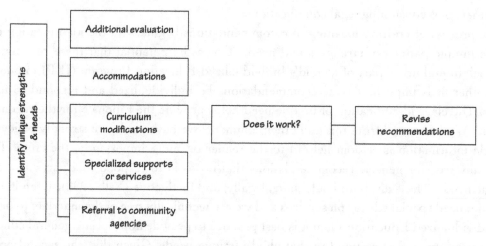

Figure 4.3   Thinking Through Recommendations

involvement of a speech-and-language pathologist or when you note fine-motor or sensory problems that might be clarified by an occupational therapy evaluation. Another version of a recommendation for further evaluation can also be the suggestion that an area assessed as part of your evaluation be reassessed at some point in the future, perhaps after providing an intervention designed to prevent an apparent weakness from growing into a bigger problem (Lichtenberger et al., 2004).

Accommodations do not require changes in the content of the curriculum but are rather designed to remove barriers and increase access to the general education curriculum. The logic of accommodations is that if a barrier is removed, the child will access the same content and material as other children. Yell (1998) divides accommodations into four categories: (1) classroom accommodations such as preferential seating; (2) academic adjustments such as allowing more time to complete an assignment, allowing a note-taker, or completing fewer items to show mastery; (3) accommodations of tests such as more time to complete a test or giving a student an exam orally rather than in writing; and (4) use of aids or technology such as a text-enlargement device. The goal here is to modify the environment so the child can access the curriculum, without fundamentally modifying the material learned.

Curriculum modifications suggest a change in what is taught or what the student is expected to learn (NICHCY, 2010). Modifications in the curriculum improve instructional match or the match between the learner's skills and the material taught (Ysseldyke & Christenson, 2002). It can involve remedial interventions or compensatory instruction that teaches needed skills but can also mean changes in structure such as providing a different level of homework or using different evaluation methods for an assignment. Remedial interventions can involve the kind of specialized instruction found in special education but might also involve academic supports in general education such as a supplemental reading program.

Supports or services can be a specialized academic program or intervention such as an individualized behavior plan or a specialized reading program but can also include any of the services regarded as related services in IDEA (IDEA, 2004). The IDEA defines related services as "services that may be required to assist the child with a disability to benefit from special education" (IDEA, §20 U.S.C. 1401 (a) (17)). The law mentions several specific services but also makes clear that this list is not exhaustive (Yell, 1998). Related services are also in the Section 504 regulations but no specific definitions are included in the statute (Yell, 1998). The services noted in IDEA are listed in Table 4.2.

A referral to a community agency or other resource might include a referral for medical evaluation or treatment or to community agencies that provide specialized psychological treatment or post-secondary transition services. Sometimes local educational agencies have contracts with agencies to provide services such as mental health treatment. Other times, community agencies provide free or low-cost services to the community.

Table 4.2   Related Services in IDEA 2004

Audiology	Parent counseling and training
Counseling	Physical therapy
Early identification and assessment	Rehabilitation counseling
Medical services	School health services
Occupational therapy	Social work services in schools
Orientation and mobility services	Speech pathology
Psychological services	Transportation
Recreation	

Connecting children and families to community resources is more difficult than it seems at first glance. We have found that this process is made easier if we frontload the parents or child with as much information as possible, including (a) name, (b) phone number, (c) address, (d) contact person, (e) appointment and intake procedures, and (f) required paperwork. Of course, not all of this information needs to be included in a written report but we have found it useful to provide this level of detail in writing at the meetings where the assessment results are discussed.

Remember, the recommendations are placed in the response to the question, "What do we need to do about this?" We have found it best to first identify a need and then offer our recommendations. Sometimes we present recommendations in a list such as the following.

Examples: Recommendations as a List

1. Max has successfully transitioned to his new school this year. He will transfer to a middle school for sixth grade this fall. To support a smooth transition and continued academic and social success, the counselor will work with Max's mother on choosing an appropriate middle school. The counselor will also contact Max's middle school counselor to share successful supports for Max.
2. Max has demonstrated excellent leadership skills and other students like him. Encouraging Max to join clubs and/or sports teams in middle school will help to continue his success with peer relationships.
3. Max has weak phonetic skills. Based on the reading assessment he needs continued instruction and practice with decoding irregular vowels and diphthongs.

In other reports, we have found it more useful to incorporate the recommendation into a narrative that responds to the "What do we need to do about this?" question.

Examples: Recommendations as a Narrative

> *Neil needs to learn to be more independent to be prepared for postsecondary life. In addition to learning to use public transportation, Neil should consider enrolling in a vocational class through the County Occupational Program. For example, the Local Occupational Program has classes in Music Technology and Careers for Children, which may fit his interests. The IEP team may also consider setting up a work internship with a special education program so that Neil can gain experience as a classroom aide.*
>
> *It may also be useful to have Neil visit local community colleges to explore their course offerings, programs, and admission processes. In addition to these activities, the IEP team should consider connecting Neil to the Department of Rehabilitation for postsecondary services.*
>
> ———
>
> *At this point, it appears that Roberto will need special education services to make adequate progress toward grade-level standards. Important areas of need include listening skills, reading, handwriting, and study skills. In reading, Roberto will benefit from a structured reading program that focuses on reading fluency and strategies for increasing reading comprehension. If possible, this should be done in addition to his regular reading program to provide additional time and practice. As mentioned earlier, if Roberto does not respond adequately to additional assistance in reading, the team should revisit the question of whether he has a learning disability. Roberto may also benefit from participation in a program such as Handwriting Without Tears. It may be useful to provide more time for all writing assignments, including note-taking, copying, and taking exams. With listening comprehension, it will be important to provide as multimodal a presentation of information as possible. Verbal instructions can be accompanied by visual cues or physical demonstrations to help Roberto focus on the verbal content. Other strategies are preferential seating near the teacher and "attention breaks," where Roberto might run an errand for the teacher, get a drink, or bring his work up to the teacher for a "check-in." Roberto might also benefit from explicit instruction in how to study and take tests. For instance, he could be taught a series of steps to go through in taking a test such as: (a) Read the test instructions before starting, (b) ask for clarification*
>
> *(continued)*

(continued)

of any instructions that you do not understand clearly, (c) look through the test to get an idea of how much you need to do in the time allowed, (d) decide how much time you should use to answer each item, (e) answer easy or known items first, then go back to the hard ones, and (f) answer all items unless there is a penalty for guessing.

⁓

Brianna needs the monitoring and support provided by a special education program. At the same time, given her cognitive and academic strengths, every effort should be made to keep her in regular classes where she can be exposed to the general curriculum. The IEP team should consider goals in the areas of attendance and work completion.

Brianna appears to have significant problems with anxiety and depression. In addition, Mrs. Gray's interview responses suggest that Brianna's most important motivations for refusing to attend school are avoidance and escape. Given this, she would likely benefit from individual or group counseling as a related service that focuses on improving her social skills, goal setting, and active problem-solving skills. Brianna may also benefit from learning and practicing a relaxation strategy such as deep breathing or progressive muscle relaxation training that would help reduce her physical symptoms of anxiety. A comprehensive anxiety treatment protocol such as "Coping Cats" may be useful in helping Brianna learn these strategies. If school-based counseling is not successful, the team should consider a referral to County Mental Health Services for a more comprehensive evaluation of her mental health needs.

⁓

Kenya is making language, social, and academic progress in her general education classroom, though she may need more one-on-one and small-group instruction to master many of the Kindergarten concepts. The team should review Kenya's Resource Specialist Program (RSP) services to determine if she needs more pull-out time to work on specific skills. Kenya can engage in work-avoidant behaviors, especially when given a non-preferred task or activity. When transitioning Kenya to her work area, do not ask her questions as a prompt, such as "Do you want to go to your work group?" Instead, give clear directions and, if needed, choices, in simple language. For example, "Kenya, it is time for small-group work. You may sit in this seat or this seat"; or "Write your name here. You may use a crayon or a pencil." If she refuses, repeat the direction, reminding her of rewards and consequences. Do not allow her to wander to a different area to do what she would rather do. Use her preferred activity as a motivation and reward for completing her work. These strategies are included in her Behavior Support Plan and should be shared with Kenya's instructional aide and the RSP aide who work with Kenya. The school psychologist and RSP teacher will collaborate with Kenya's team to make sure all team members are using consistent language and rewards/consequences when working with Kenya.

TRY IT!

DEVELOP RECOMMENDATIONS

Using information from one of your reports, consider three unique needs that you identified in your evaluation. For each one, consider what an appropriate recommendation might be using the categories discussed in this chapter.

UNIQUE NEED	ADDITIONAL EVALUATION	ACCOMMODATION	MODIFICATION	SERVICE	REFERRAL
1.					
2.					
3.					

To summarize this section, we recommend that you always offer meaningful recommendations, link them clearly to unique needs, and consider the child's needs for each of the following types of recommendations of (a) additional evaluation, (b) accommodations, (c) instructional or curriculum modifications, (d) specialized supports or services, and (e) referrals to a community agency or other resource.

Chapter 4 Takeaway Points

- There should be logical connections between each aspect of the evaluation, including the reason for referral, evaluation questions, procedures chosen to conduct the evaluation results, and the recommendations that follow from the evaluation.
- The Reason for Referral section of the report communicates the background and rationale for the evaluation.
- Most evaluations will have three types of questions: (1) current levels of functioning questions, (2) disability or diagnostic questions, and (3) recommendations or "What do we need to do differently?" questions.
- The background information provides sufficient information about children to situate them in a developmental, social, and educational context and the factors that might play a role in explaining the concerns raised by the report consumers.
- In question-driven, referral-based reports the interpretation and integration of assessment data is *not* left to the Conclusion or Summary section, but rather, it is ongoing and explicit and presented as an answer to the evaluation questions.
- Assessment data from multiple sources are integrated into themes to answer each evaluation question.
- Meaningful recommendations are student specific and clearly explained, directly tied to the assessment results, and reflect an understanding of the classroom environment and the curriculum.
- Always offer meaningful recommendations. Even if a child does not need special education services and we are technically free of the mandate to develop an Individualized Education Plan, it is best practice to provide appropriate general education recommendations that respond to that child's unique needs.

CHAPTER 5

How Do I Solve Practical Problems Along the Way to Question-Driven Report Writing?

Neither of us began our journey to become better report writers using the questions-driven referral-based format we currently advocate. Our progression is the result of years of teaching, research, reading, reflection, and rebuilding. This development is a dynamic process and we continue to modify and fine-tune our writing styles in the pursuit of a useful report.

Our final chapter is designed to provide specific strategies for solving problems and smoothing the transition to a new writing style. For many of our readers, you may have been using the same report structure or template for years. However, we hope that we have fostered a desire to give your reports a more useful purpose and provided clear steps on how to reach this goal. Change can be difficult, and in adopting this report-writing model you are also adopting a different way of addressing your evaluations. You are embracing the fact that report writing is an integral part of the assessment process and accepting the ethical and legal responsibility to make your reports more useful for your consumers. We applaud you for wanting to take that step.

This chapter is organized around frequently asked questions we receive from both students and professionals as they transition to a question-driven, referral-based report writing style. We have also included some summary questions to remind you of key themes in the book.

REMIND ME: WHY IS ANOTHER BOOK ON REPORT WRITING NEEDED?

This was the title of Chapter 1. Multiple books on the market explain *how* to write a psychoeducational or psychological report. Our book is distinctly different. We do give guidelines and recommendations on how to structure and write your report, but all of these have a fundamental goal. We strive to write useful and accessible psychoeducational reports that through their structure and underlying philosophy are legally defensible. This book presents not just how to do this but *why* you should aim for a useful report and how a useful report is more ethical and easy to legally defend.

IDEA (2004) provides clear guidelines regarding parents' right to be involved in the evaluation process and to participate in the decisions that follow. Parents need to be provided information they can understand if they are to be authentically informed participants in their child's educational planning and decision making. The ethical and legal obligation to ensure that parents have access to the information they need to authentically and fully participate in the evaluation and decision-making process falls on us as professionals. To be useful for consumers and to make this participation less complicated for consumers, our reports need to clearly answer the referral questions, focus on strengths as well as needs, provide concrete and feasible recommendations for educational planning, and be written so that they are clear and understandable.

WHY SHOULD I CHANGE MY REPORT WRITING MODEL?

Bluntly put, the answer to this question is "to be more useful." Most school psychologists engage in assessment-related activities more than all other activities combined, though many of us have lost our way in a swamp of poorly constructed templates and professional jargon (yes, we know this is dramatic) and are engaging in report writing that does not have a clear purpose in mind. Well-conceptualized assessment practices and effective psychoeducational reports can shape the value and relevance of our services. The psychological report is a direct reflection of the quality and range of services school psychologists provide. They also provide us with reassurance that our practice is legally sound, when questions or concerns do arise.

Assessments and reports framed by collaborative consultation, assessment-based answers to referral questions, and quality recommendations exemplify our ability to engage in a broader range of school psychological services. Through the use of an assessment and report writing model such as question-driven referral-based, our expertise in assessment can be the leverage for more active and useful involvement in collaboration, consultation, prevention, and intervention.

What Should Be My First Steps Toward Transitioning to This Report Style?

As we have previously stated, report writing is an integral but often-overlooked part of the assessment process. We assume that your goal in adopting this format is to write more useful reports. Regardless of the format used, you *cannot* write a useful report from a poorly conducted assessment. So, our first step is for you to critically look at your assessment practices to make sure you are gathering useful data and information. Refer back to Figure 4.1 (Chapter 4), which illustrates our view of the evaluation cycle. If we were to think about adopting these practices developmentally, we would suggest the following sequence:

1. Start with developing evaluation questions. If you are using a traditional format with a summary or conclusion section, at least address them there.
2. Strengthen your Reason for Referral section. Try to add detail that is unique to the child and expresses the concerns raised by the referring parties.
3. Try using your evaluation questions as headings and integrate data to answer those questions.
4. At logical places in your narrative, try using theme statements as subheadings.

In the following section, we will address how to integrate this model into a preexisting template.

My School District or Agency Already Has a Template That We Are Required to Use; How Can I Work Within These Constraints?

This is one of the most common questions we receive from our students in their fieldwork and from professionals who attend our trainings. It is not uncommon for school districts to create a structured template for their school psychologists to use when writing reports. This is sometimes done for consistency so that reports look similar across all of the service providers in the district. We don't disagree with this strategy; we simply believe that many of these templates do not lend themselves to consumer usefulness. Strict templates can also begin to guide your assessment practices, where the idea of an individualized assessment is lost among the template structure. The report headings start to impact what we assess, how we assess, and how we describe results, leading our reports to look strikingly similar for every student. Unfortunately, school districts also create templates as a legally defensive measure. These are the templates we discussed in Chapter 2, where there is heavy use of boilerplate legal language. Inclusion of statements that inform the reader of the legal mandates for the assessment or quotations taken directly from legal documents bestows a false sense of protection. Remember, writing it does not make it true. The accuracy of these statements needs to be evident to the reader. It is the responsibility of the report writer to show the reader that these mandates have been met rather than simply telling them.

In many of the conversations we have had with practitioners, we realized that rarely do school psychologists question the use of a set template in their district. They accept the template as status quo. However, when their administrators or lead psychologists are approached with a new writing format, examples of what this might look like, and most importantly, the evidence that this style is more useful and legally defensible, they are often more open to change than expected. So our first advice is for practitioners in districts with a set report writing template to approach their administrator with the goal of improving the usefulness of their reports for consumers and more efficiently meeting legal mandates. Provide one of our examples and then also one that you have prepared.

There are definitely school districts that are not going to be easily swayed by the rational presentation of the benefits of this assessment and writing style. In our experience, these tend to be school districts engaged in a great deal of Special Education litigation that have paid legal teams, not educators or psychologists, to create a "legally defensible" writing template. These reports often become compliance documents that are very difficult to read, rather than useful communication tools. Remember, the goal of our assessment is to assist with educational planning and positively influence consumers' (i.e., teachers' and parents') interactions with the student. The report documents students' present levels of performance and educational needs and is the foundation of the IEP. To be useful for consumers, our reports need to clearly answer the referral questions, focus on strengths as well as needs, provide concrete and feasible recommendations for educational planning, and be written so that they are clear and understandable.

Most district-created templates are a mix of domain- and test-based structures. Let us quickly review why we do not recommend the use of test-based or domain-based report structures and then we will address each of these concerns. First, both of these styles can lead to a strict use of test or domain headings that can predetermine assessment areas and/or tools. Second, this style of presentation lends itself to very limited integration of assessment data. The reader usually has to wade through multiple pages of test descriptions and results before a summary, while trying understand and integrate multiple sources of data.

If you must use a district-created template, our first piece of advice is to separate the template from your assessment practices. Your district's template basically becomes an organizational structure. Do not let the template frame your evaluation or limit your assessment choices and outcomes. Remember that the written report is a vital part of the assessment process, not a post-assessment obligation. Once the reason(s) for referral have been identified, the referral questions guide your evaluation, including the assessment tools you choose, how you interpret the assessment data, and how you develop your results into meaningful recommendations.

Our second piece of advice is to focus on making your reports more readable. Use the strategies we provide in Chapter 3 to make the writing in your report clearer and more understandable to your readers.

1. Reduce professional jargon by eliminating technical terminology or defining these terms using simpler vocabulary and specific behavioral examples.
2. Consider the length of your reports, including the amount and quality of information you include.
3. Focus the report on information about a particular child and reduce the amount of generic information.
4. Do not take it for granted that your terminology or tables are self-explanatory.
5. Take the time to provide clearly worded definitions and student-specific examples of what abstract constructs may look like at home or at school.
6. If you must include detailed information about specific tests or tables, we recommend that you move them to appendixes.

Finally, refer back to the developmental sequence provided in the previous question. Start with developing evaluation questions. If you are using a traditional format with a summary or conclusion section, at least address them there. Strengthen your Reason for Referral section. Try to add detail that is unique to this child and expresses the concerns raised by the referring parties.

Within your report narrative ensure that you integrate data from multiple data sources, highlight relevant findings, and develop quality recommendations. This may seem to be a challenge in test or domain-based templates, but it is possible. We encourage the use of questions or explanatory statements connected to the headings of forced templates. For example, under the heading Cognitive Abilities, a short question or statement is provided that explains the purpose of this section, such as, *Cynthia's cognitive abilities were assessed using data from a review of her school records, parent and teacher interviews and the Differential Ability Scales–2. In this section we answer the questions: What are Cynthia's cognitive processing strengths and weaknesses? How do these strengths and weaknesses impact her learning?*

This statement provides a context for the information that will follow and encourages the writer to integrate data from multiple sources into relevant and informative findings. At the end of the section, provide an integrated summary answering the two questions (*In this section we answer the questions: What are Cynthia's cognitive processing strengths and weaknesses? How do these strengths and weaknesses impact her learning? Based on the data collected . . .*).

Use these strategies to include an introductory purpose and summary of data after each domain or test heading so that information from all sources (i.e., reviews of records, interviews, observations, and testing) can be integrated. When these summaries are provided after each section of the template, they will help guide the reader through the assessment and written report. Example 5 in Appendix II uses a domain-based structure, though it follows a referral-based model of evaluation.

This Style of Report Writing Seems Time Consuming and I Am Already Swamped with Work! Is This True?

After the template question, this is the second-most-common question we receive. We don't agree that this style of report writing is more time consuming, though it will be when you first begin. Any time we learn something new and incorporate it into our everyday practice, it takes extra time. For example, as students and new psychologists you probably spend hours more on reports than you do as experienced school psychologists. The transition here will be no different. Your first few reports will be more time consuming, but once you start to get the hang of it, we think the overall process is more efficient and it becomes less time consuming in the writing and in the presentation of results to the IEP team.

You are a trained school psychologist, not a diagnostician or assessment technician. As a school psychologist, it is your responsibility to interpret the data, not simply report it, and then integrate the data into meaningful results. If this sounds challenging, then the transition process may be longer because you are going to need to reframe your role in the assessment process from passive (filling in blanks in a template with your assessment data) to active (having your report structure serve you as a useful way to present your evaluation results). If you are already interpreting and integrating data from multiple sources, then the transition to a referral-based report will be much easier.

Out time is precious. As practicing psychologists, we are both very aware of the time limitations placed on school psychologists. We both practice in a state where budget woes have significantly increased caseloads while simultaneously decreasing time at our school sites. We need to use our time more effectively and efficiently. Look back at Figure 4.1, "Evaluation Cycle," in Chapter 4. Where do you believe you spend the most time in the evaluation process? We think most school psychologists spend the majority of their time conducting testing during the Conduct Assessments stage. Although this is clearly a vital part of the evaluation cycle, to engage in a question-driven, referral-based assessment and report you will need to reorganize your assessment time allocation. More time is spent during the early stages of the cycle, including clarifying concerns and the reason for referral, designing questions and hypotheses, and choosing assessment procedures and tools. We hope it is implicit what this means you won't be doing. We don't mean to be patronizing, but to be clear: This means you will not send an Assessment Plan home before speaking with the parent and teacher and reviewing the students' records. You will not automatically assess in every area possible and you will not use the same battery of tests for each student.

It is important to develop an accurate list of concerns early in the evaluation process. This provides a focus for your evaluation questions and informs your choice of assessment procedures. Although it is always possible to discover something about a child you did not suspect going into an evaluation, it is our experience that most often it is feasible and practical to narrow the suspected disabilities to a small number of possibilities. Sharpening the focus of your evaluation clarifies the entire evaluation process and prevents us from over-assessing children, making the assessment process less intrusive for children and teachers. It simultaneously saves us time and makes for a more coherent and efficiently conducted assessment. Surely this is a win-win for everyone involved.

DO REFERRAL-BASED REPORTS VARY, DEPENDING ON THE CHARACTERISTICS OF THE CHILD?

The answer to this question is, "yes and no." The basic structure will not change, but the questions we ask and the nature of the information we gather will likely vary. For example, if we were assessing a child who is bilingual, we would ask questions about language use and preference. We would also be interested in the child's level of language development in both English and his or her home language. This information would likely go into the Background section, although we might also pose specific evaluation questions such as "How well can Lina speak English and Spanish?" or "What language does Lina speak best?" or "What language or languages will provide the most accurate information regarding Lina's abilities?" In addition, there are few appropriate standardized tests for use with bilingual youth, so most evaluations will focus on the *RIO* (records, interviews, and observations) aspect of the RIOT framework and less on the *T* (test). This will mean the report will contain more descriptive narrative than you would find in an evaluation with a monolingual, English-speaking child.

The answer is similar for evaluations done with children with different suspected disabilities. Our experience is that evaluations focused on certain disabilities (e.g., emotional disturbance, or Other Health Impaired) also will have more RIO and less T. Several of our examples in Appendix II focus on these issues and hopefully you will find them helpful.

DO TRIENNIAL REEVALUATIONS DIFFER FROM OTHER REPORTS?

The answer is again, "yes and no." As with characteristics of the child, the basic structure and ideas behind the assessment do not change. Nevertheless, because our evaluations and reports are individualized, they will of course differ. *Triennials*, or three-year reevaluations, have a legal purpose. They are designed to evaluate whether the student's eligibility, place-ment, and services are meeting their educational needs. Given that, we have found certain things helpful with reevaluations.

As with all our reports, we write an expanded Reason for Referral section. In this section we note how long the child has been in special education, what his current disability clas-sification is, what services he receives, and what, if any, new concerns are present. See the example of Christy in what follows.

Example: Triennial Reason for Referral

> *Christy has received special education services since Kindergarten. When she was first evaluated, she was identified as a student with a "developmental delay." In first grade, her special education classification was changed to "specific learning dis-ability." In eighth grade, Christy was reevaluated and her classification was again changed to "speech and language impairment."*
>
> *Christy currently attends Local High School where she is enrolled in a combi-nation of general education classes, general education classes with push-in spe-cial education support, and special education classes. Her current Individualized Education Plan (IEP) has goals in reading comprehension, written expression, vocabulary, math calculation, and organizational skills.*
>
> *When interviewed, Christy's mom said that she has concerns about her short-term memory and her performance in math. In math, she says Christy has trouble remembering steps and procedures to solve math problems.*

Note how this is similar to our general recommendations for a Reason for Referral section. We know enough about Christy to understand better the focus of this evaluation beyond meet-ing a vague legal requirement. The questions that follow are also similar but phrased somewhat differently. For example, the disability question could be phrased as "Does Christy continue to have a speech and language impairment?" and the "What do we do about it" question may become "What, if any, additions or modifications to Christy's special education and related services are needed to enable her to meet the annual goals in her individualized education program?"

Of course, some reevaluations are straightforward and require little, if any, formal evaluation beyond a through record review. Others will require more extensive formal evaluation. As with all evaluations, this will be driven by the nature of the concerns and the evaluation questions that follow from those concerns. A full example of a triennial evaluation is included in Appendix II.

HOW DO CHARTS AND TABLES FIT INTO A QUESTIONS-BASED THEMATIC REPORT?

As with an academic article or technical writing of any sort, charts, tables, or figures should be used to help the reader better understand complex information. Keeping this in mind, when you consider whether to insert a chart or table into a report, it is important to ask yourself if that chart or table will be truly helpful to the reader. In many of the reports we read, each test or behavior rating scale is followed by a table listing all of the scores for each index, subtest, or scale. Even as experienced professionals, we find all these data overwhelming. It can also lead to inappropriate interpretations by less knowledgeable readers. (Yes, Jeanne Anne once had to spend a significant amount of time explaining to a lawyer why a single subtest scale score of 6 did not equate to a learning disability!) It is easy to imagine that parents or teachers will rarely find this "throwing data on the page" strategy to be useful. After all, it is our responsibility as professionals to give meaning to these data, and not simply report them, leaving the interpretation to the reader. If you believe this type of data is potentially helpful to a reader, then we recommend you place the charts or tables as appendixes so they will not interrupt the flow of the narrative of the report.

One way to think about this is to ask the question, "Will this chart or table do a better job of explaining the meaning of these data than I can do in a narrative?" Some examples include using a table to organize a complex school history where a child has changed schools often. In this case, it is often confusing to read a listing of several schools in a paragraph and it is clearer to read them in a chronological list or a table format. We have also used tables to represent progress-monitoring data, such as the type of information that might be gathered during an academic response-to-intervention process or a behavior plan. In this case, a graph with an upward- or downward-sloping trend-line will often be a much more powerful communication of progress than a narrative explaining that progress. Of course, in each of these cases, these visual aids should be accompanied by a short narrative explaining them and highlighting the findings. It is the combination of words and a visual representation that makes these strong representations of the point being made.

Do I Need to Use a Specific Format When Writing?

This is really up to the writer, though we cannot emphasize enough that you need to be consistent in how you choose to format your report. For example, we often see reports where each table, chart, and heading is formatted differently. This simply becomes a confusing visual mess for the reader. We recommend that you consider using the general guidelines for layout and formatting described by the *Publication Manual of the American Psychological Association, Sixth Edition* (American Psychological Association, 2006). These include margins, page numbering, font, headings, subheadings, and even tables and charts. Many reports have a running head of some sort and we recommend that if you use one, you also format that according to APA style.

There are two main reasons for recommending that you use APA formatting and layout conventions. The first is that most practitioners are familiar with APA style from graduate school. Thus, you do not have to learn something new or, worse yet, make something up. The second reason is that it will ultimately make your life as a report writer easier. Once you have settled on a format, you can build this into a template and, for the most part, forget about it. The purpose of formatting and layout conventions is to make reading a paper or report easier for the reader. It also communicates that you are familiar with the conventions of your profession or, put another way, you have the knowledge and background to write like a psychologist.

Formatting, especially the use of subheadings and tables, is meant to make the report easier to read. Many of the psychoeducational reports we have read have very complicated formatting, especially in their use of subheadings and tables. From our point of view, this makes them more difficult rather than easier to read for almost all of the potential consumers of the report. It is obvious from reading these reports that the authors made formatting choices that made things easier for themselves as writers rather than for the reader. Good reports, like good writing of any sort, are reader centered rather than author centered. As we have stated before, when considering whether to use tables or charts or how many subheadings to use, consider whether they are truly helpful for the consumer.

Last Words

In the appendixes that follow this final chapter, we have included seven different report samples as well as a checklist to use to evaluate your current reports. You will note that the sample reports are different, both stylistically and in terms of the characteristics of the children involved. We do this purposefully so you can choose how to implement the suggestions we offer in your own way.

Last Words

We do not underestimate the challenge of shifting your perspective on reports and implementing a set of new strategies. At the same time, we urge you to make the effort. We do not believe you need to implement everything we have reviewed, especially all at once. Yet, we also believe that implementing some of the suggestions we have made will improve your practice. One of the points we have tried to make is that you cannot separate the evaluation process from how you write your reports. Given this, we think that changing how you write your reports will change how you view your evaluations and even how you view the children you work with. This is a good thing. Our reports are a direct reflection of the quality and range of services we can provide as school psychologists. We contend that our reports should reflect the dynamic nature of the problem-solving process and serve as a foundation for engaging in more consultation, prevention, and intervention. A referral-based, question-driven model of assessment and report writing can be an important tool in your journey to expand your scope of practice and make your services more useful to parents, teachers, and other educators.

We assume that if you are reading this last paragraph, you have made the considerable effort to read this book and are ready to begin this process. As one of our good friends and colleagues often says: *Onward!*

Checklist for a Useful and Legally Defensible Report

We have created a checklist to help you evaluate whether your reports are useful and legally defensible. Our checklist reflects the key recommendations and guidelines from Chapters 1 through 5. We have divided it into the following sections: Evaluation Planning, Report Sections, Writing Strategies, and Useful and Legally Defensible.

AREA		✔	CONCEPT
Evaluation Planning			I consulted with the referring party (parents and teachers) to identify areas of concern and clarify the referral questions.
			From the concerns, I identified clear evaluation questions.
			I collaborated with the referring party (parents and teachers) to create the Assessment Plan, choosing tools that gather data that will directly answer the evaluation questions.
			I chose a variety of evaluation tools and procedures (i.e., RIOT & Rule of Two).
			I chose evaluation tools that provided relevant data that will help parents and teachers who work with the student.
			I chose evaluation tools that collected functional data grounded in real life.
			The tools and procedures I used were reliable and valid.
			The tools I used were not racially or culturally biased and were chosen to yield accurate information about the child, given his or her language, culture, and limitations in sensory, motor, and speaking skills.
Report	*Reason for Referral*		I clearly communicated the rationale for the evaluation, including concerns, the recent history of the problem, and symptoms or behaviors that led to the referral.
			I clearly stated what areas or domains are to be assessed.
			I clearly stated what disabilities are suspected.
Report	*Evaluation Questions*		My evaluation included current levels of functioning questions.
			My evaluation included disability or diagnostic questions.
			My evaluation included "What do we need to do differently?" questions.
Report	*Background History*		The background information provided sufficient information about children to situate them in a developmental, social, and educational context.
			The background information included factors that might play a role in explaining the concerns raised by the referring party.

AREA	✓	CONCEPT
Report / *Evaluation Results*		I interpreted assessment data from multiple sources in the context of the referral questions.
		When presenting evaluation results, I used themes as headings or thematic statements to answer each evaluation question.
		The interpretation and integration of assessment data was not left to the Conclusion or Summary section, but rather, was ongoing and explicit.
		I clearly included information on the student's strengths as well as needs.
		I clearly answered the referral questions.
Report / *Recommendations*		My recommendations are directly tied to the assessment results.
		My recommendations are student specific rather than generic.
		My recommendations are clearly explained so that a teacher or school team will know how to carry them out.
		My recommendations reflect an understanding of the classroom environment and the curriculum.
Writing Strategies		I removed boilerplate legal language from my report and showed, rather than told, the reader that my evaluation met legal guidelines.
		I reduced the professional jargon in my report or provided clear behavioral examples of technical terms.
		I decreased the length of my report by removing generic statements and cutting excess words.
		I wrote with an active, rather than passive voice, as much as possible.
		I used a report structure (e.g., questions and themes) that integrates data and highlights relevant evaluation findings.

AREA		✔	CONCEPT
Useful & Legally Defensible Evaluation			There is a logical connection between each aspect of the evaluation, including (a) the reason for referral, (b) evaluation questions, (c) procedures chosen to conduct the evaluation, and (d) the recommendations that follow from the evaluation results.
			I assessed in all areas of suspected disability.
			I assessed in all areas of suspected need.
			My evaluation helps consumers understand the child better, including determining a diagnosis or disability classification.
			My evaluation provides information that helps consumers work more effectively with this child.
			My evaluation provides information that directly leads to interventions and/or accommodations.
			My evaluation included functional information grounded in real-life contexts.
			My evaluation was fair. The tools I used were not racially or culturally biased and were chosen to yield accurate information about the child, given his or her language, culture, and limitations in sensory, motor, and speaking skills.
			I have conducted an evaluation within my scope of practice and experience.
			I support all IEP team members' active participation by giving copies of my report to the team members prior to the meeting so they could read and process the information prior to making educational decisions about the student.

What Do These Reports Look Like?

In this appendix, we provide six different examples of reports using a *question-driven, referral-based* report model. The first thing you may notice is that although they all use the same model, they also look different from each other. This is because there are two different authors who have both implemented this model in their own ways and writing styles. For example, Michael tends to write about the assessment tools he chooses in statements, where Jeanne Anne uses a list organized around the RIOT model. In Jeanne Anne's reports, she includes an italicized and bolded answer to the evaluation question directly after the question, and then provides the narrative of how she got to this answer, whereas Michael usually uses thematic statements throughout the narrative to answer evaluation questions. Please note, these are simply personal writing differences and the key elements of the report writing style are all intact. We have purposefully selected reports that represent children of different ages and Special Education eligibilities as well as reports that have slightly different formats and styles. All of them are consistent with the approach we advocate but offer options for your consideration. We want to remind you that we have changed all identifying information to preserve the confidentiality of the children, parents, teachers, and other professionals we mention in these samples.

Example 1: High School Student, Reevaluation
Assessing for Intellectual Disability

This report is written at a 12.1 Flesch Kincaid grade level with 16% passive sentences.

Name: Mike Stewart
Chronological Age: 17-3

Reason for Referral and Assessment Questions:
Mike's mother referred him for an evaluation. He has received special education services since Kindergarten. He was eligible for special education services as a student with a "developmental delay" until May of DATE, when his special education classification was changed to "specific learning disability." In eighth grade, Mike was reevaluated and his classification was again changed to "speech and language impairment." Mike currently attends Local City High School where he is enrolled in a combination of general education classes, general education classes with push-in special education support, and special education classes. His current Individualized Education Plan (IEP) has goals in reading comprehension, written expression, vocabulary, algebra, math calculation, auditory processing, figurative language, and organization.

When interviewed, Mrs. Stewart said that Mike's "cognitive levels are low." She was also concerned about his short-term memory and his performance in math. In math, she says he has trouble remembering steps and procedures to solve math problems.

This assessment is being conducted to answer the following questions:

1. What are Mike's current levels of intellectual and academic development?
2. How well developed are Mike's adaptive skills? For example, how independent is he at home and in the community?
3. What is Mike's current level of social and emotional development?
4. What is the most appropriate educational diagnosis or classification for Mike?
5. What changes, if any, are needed in Mike's Individualized Education Plan for him to make adequate progress toward district and state academic standards?
6. What changes, if any, are needed in Mike's Transition Plan for him to achieve his post-secondary goals?

Assessment Procedures:
1. Review of school records, including prior assessment reports from the school district as well as a local mental health clinic.

2. Mrs. Stewart was interviewed on 1/17/DATE, 1/27/DATE, and 2/17/DATE. On 1/27/DATE, Mrs. Stewart was interviewed using the *Vineland-II Adaptive Behavior Scales Survey Interview* form. Mrs. Stewart also completed the *Behavior System for Children–3, Structured Developmental History,* and the *Social Skill Improvement System Rating Scale.*

3. Mike was interviewed on 1/27/DATE, 2/13/DATE, and 2/27/DATE. On 2/13/DATE, he completed the *Kaufman Assessment Battery for Children II, Non-Verbal Index.* On 2/27/DATE, he also completed the *Social Skills Improvement System Rating Scale.*

4. Mrs. Hass, Michael's Speech and Language Therapist, was interviewed on 1/27/DATE. Mrs. Hass also completed the *Vineland-II Adaptive Behavior Scale* and the teacher version of the *Social Skills Improvement System Rating Scale.*

5. Mr. Smith, Mike's Life Science teacher, completed the teacher version of the *Social Skills Improvement System Rating Scale* on 2/26/DATE.

Background Information and Record Review:

Background information about Mike was obtained from a review of his school records and Mrs. Stewart's responses to questions on the *Behavioral Assessment for Children–3, Structured Developmental History* (BASC-3 SDH), which she completed as part of this evaluation.

Mike is an only child who lives at home with his mother and stepfather. Mrs. Stewart separated from Mike's biological father when he was about nine months old. When interviewed, Mike said he does not see his biological father and described him as "out of the picture." Mrs. Stewart and Mike's stepfather have been together for about 12 years.

Mrs. Stewart was healthy during her pregnancy with Mike and she and Mike were healthy at his birth. Mike appears to have met his early developmental milestones within typical time periods. For example, he stood alone at 9 months, walked at 10 months, spoke first words at 1 year, and spoke in sentences at 2 years.

Mike has scoliosis of the spine but this does not cause him pain or limit his physical activity. Mike is currently healthy and has normal vision and hearing. Although his vision and hearing are normal, Mike has been identified as having deficits in both visual and auditory processing.

In December 2004, Mike was assessed at a private speech-and-language therapist. A report of this evaluation describes Mike as having deficits in several areas of auditory processing and recommends the use of a personal FM monitoring system. According to Mrs. Stewart, Mike used an FM monitor to assist with auditory processing until it was "faded" in high school.

Tom Hathaway, Vision Specialist, also assessed Mike in December of DATE to determine if he had a visual processing deficit. Mr. Hathaway's report describes Mike as having good visual acuity and normal "basic eye functions." The report also describes Mike as having visual processing deficits and recommends several classroom accommodations. A vision progress report written by Mr. Hathaway and dated 1/27/DATE recommends that Mike be dismissed from the "vision consultation program."

In April of DATE, Jim Brady, MD, assessed Mike. Dr. Brady's report notes that Mike was doing well socially at the time but goes on to describe him as having a "very unusual form of high-functioning autism." Dr. Brady also notes a history of having difficulty with transitions, sensitivity to loud sounds, and an "affinity" to textures.

As noted above, Mike has received special education services since Kindergarten. At different times since then, he has been classified as a student with a developmental delay, a learning disability, and a speech and language impairment. Autism and intellectual disability have also been considered as possible educational diagnoses but have been ruled out by prior evaluations. Mike received special education services in a special day class from first through eighth grade. He was retained in the fifth grade. Mrs. Stewart notes in the BASC-3 SDH that at the time, she did not believe that Mike was mature enough for middle school.

As noted above, Mike is currently enrolled at Local City High School in a combination of general education classes, general education classes with push-in special education support, and special education classes.

Responses to Assessment Questions: The information below is organized by the assessment questions listed above. In the response to each question, the italicized statements in the text boxes are summaries or theme statements. Supporting information is in the text that follows each statement.

What are Mike's current levels of intellectual and academic development?

> *Mike's academic development is mixed. He is currently earning A's and B's in all of his classes, including his general education classes of Life Science and Guitar. His academic skills, as measured by the Woodcock Johnson IV Tests of Achievement, are in the low to low-average range and his performance on state testing is "far below basic" in Algebra, English–Language Arts, Life Science, and World History. He has not yet passed the high school exit exam.*

Appendix II

Mike's 3/16/DATE Individualized Education Program (IEP) has goals in reading comprehension, written expression, vocabulary, algebra, math calculation, auditory processing, figurative language, and organization. Mike is currently enrolled in special education for history and study skills. He is enrolled in a collaborative English class, where special education support is available in the general education class. In addition, Mike takes general education classes in guitar and life science. He also receives 45 minutes weekly of speech and language therapy.

A report card dated 1/27/DATE shows Mike as earning two A's and three B's. His English and Study Skills teachers both comment that he is a pleasure to have in class. Mike has twice taken, but not passed, the High School Exit Exam. At the time of his last state testing in May of DATE, Mike earned scores that were described "far below basic" in Algebra, English-Language Arts, Life Science, and World History.

As part of his three-year reevaluation in November and December of DATE, Mike was given the *Woodcock Johnson IV Tests of Achievement* (WJ IV ACH). Mike's performance in reading, written language, and math generally fell in the range of scores considered low to low-average. For example, he earned a standard score of 85 in Broad Reading, a standard score of 82 in Broad Written Language, and a standard score of 81 in Broad Math.

Mike's global intellectual abilities have been assessed several times with different standardized tests. He has consistently scored in the range of scores considered low to very low.

Mike's intellectual abilities have been assessed eight times since DATE using the *Kaufman Assessment Battery for Children, Kaufman Assessment Battery for Children II,* the *Stanford Binet IV,* the *Wechsler Intelligence Scale for Children IV,* and the *Wechsler Adult Intelligence Scale IV.* His performance on the *Stanford Binet IV*, administered when he was in Kindergarten, was average. The other seven times his intellectual abilities were assessed, his scores were consistently below average, ranging from a standard score of 67 to a standard score of 74. In addition, Mike's performances across the various cognitive abilities assessed by these tests have been consistent. The one exception to this was the recent administration in December of DATE of the *Wechsler Adult Intelligence Scale IV* by Western Youth Services. In this case, Mike's verbal skills as measured by the Verbal Comprehension Index fell in the low-average range while his other scores, including the full scale IQ, were below average, ranging between standard scores of 71 and 76.

Given Mike's history of difficulties with oral language, as part of this evaluation he was given the *Kaufman Assessment Battery for Children II, Nonverbal Index*

(KABC II NVI). The KABC II NVI assesses intellectual ability by using tests that do not require verbal expression and use only simple verbal instructions.

Mike's performance on the KABC II NVI was also significantly below average. His standard score of 72 is similar to his performance on prior assessments of his intellectual ability.

How well developed are Mike's adaptive skills? For example, how independent is he at home and in the community?

> *There are significant differences between Mike's independence at home and at school. At home and in the community, Mike seems much less independent than typical for someone his age. At school, Mike's adaptive behavior appears more typical.*

As part of this evaluation, Mrs. Stewart was interviewed regarding Mike's adaptive behavior using the *Vineland II Adaptive Behavior Scales Survey Interview* form. In addition, Mrs. Hass, Michael's Speech and Language Therapist, completed the *Vineland II Adaptive Behavior Scales Teacher Rating* form.

Adaptive behavior can be defined as the ability to cope with everyday demands and includes the skills persons use to take care of themselves and relate to others. On the Vineland II, this includes communication skills, daily living skills, and social skills. Performance on the Vineland II is described as adequate, moderately low, or low. These classifications are based on comparisons with other persons the same age as Mike.

Mike's mother appears to view him as being much less independent than other 17-year-olds. Her responses to the Vineland II fall in the range of scores considered low or moderately low. This represents standard scores of 68 in daily living skills, 74 in communication skills, and 76 in socialization.

Mrs. Stewart views Mike as more dependent on routines and parent prompting than is typical for students his age. She says that although Mike can hold a conversation for at least 10 minutes, he has difficulty explaining ideas in more than one way or giving directions to others. He can care for his own basic grooming but does not always choose clothes appropriate for the weather. He washes his own clothes on family "laundry day" but does not use a stove or oven to cook without supervision. Mike uses the phone appropriately but cannot use public transportation.

In contrast to Mrs. Stewart's perceptions of Mike at home, Mrs. Hass appears to see Mike has having typical adaptive behavior skills. Her scores on the teacher version of the Vineland fell in the "adequate" range. Her responses resulted in standard scores of 94 in daily living skill, 93 in communication, and 103 in socialization.

Mike's current Individual Transition Plan, which was developed at the time of his last IEP on 1/16/DATE, notes that he wants to seek training to work in a music store and live independently. The transition plan notes that Mike wants to play guitar in a band. Recommended activities include researching employment opportunities, developing self-advocacy skills, and developing a budget for living expenses.

What is Mike's current level of social and emotional development?

During the assessment, Mike was cooperative and did not show obvious signs of anxiety or depression. He has goals for the future and enjoys music and playing the guitar. Mike reports friends outside of school and views himself as having typical social skills. Despite this, he seems to have limited social interactions at school.

Mike was interviewed on 1/27, 2/13, and 2/27/DATE. On 2/13/DATE, Mike also completed the *Social Skills Improvement System Rating Scales* (SSIS). During the initial interview, Mike was cooperative and responded to questions openly. Mike views himself as doing well in his classes but believes he needs more help in math. Mike talked about seeing a therapist this past summer because he needed to learn about "communicating better." He said he thought therapy was helpful at first, but after a while, he felt he no longer needed it.

Mike enjoys music and playing the guitar. At home, he reports doing chores and homework and playing the guitar. When asked about his goals, Mike said he wanted to live on his own and work in a music store.

A report of an evaluation conducted by Local Mental Health Clinic in December of DATE says that Mike presented with "flat affect and his mood was unusually apathetic, irritable, anxious, or depressed." During the three interviews conducted as part of this evaluation, Mike did not express a wide range of emotions but also did not seem unusually anxious, sad, or irritable. When interviewed as part of this evaluation, Mike did say that sometimes he does not sleep well because his "mind races." Mike talked about visiting friends outside of school but said that at lunch he mostly walks around and "says hi" to people.

The SSIS Rating Scales assesses a variety of positive social skills such as sharing, helping others, and controlling one's temper. These positive social skills are organized into seven areas or subscales: Communication, Cooperation, Assertion, Responsibility, Empathy, Engagement, and Self-Control. Scores in these areas are described as Below Average, Average, and Above Average. A Below Average behavior level indicates that the individual may need assistance to improve the skills in that area. The SSIS Rating Scale also assesses negative or maladaptive behaviors such as externalizing behaviors (e.g., aggression, acting out), bullying, hyperactivity/inattention, internalizing problems (e.g., depression, anxiety, withdrawal), and behaviors associated with the autism spectrum.

Mike's responses to the SSIS suggest he sees himself as having above-average positive social skills and average levels of maladaptive or problem behaviors.

Mrs. Stewart does not see Mike as anxious or depressed. She views him as having average basic social skills but notes problems with turn-taking and eye contact. She also notes problems with acting without thinking, being easily distracted, and becoming upset when his routine changed.

When Mrs. Stewart was interviewed, she said that she did not believe Mike was anxious or depressed. She views him as fitting in socially but also sees him as having difficulty making social judgments. Mrs. Stewart completed the parent version of the SSIS Rating Scale. Her responses to the SSIS suggest that overall, she sees Mike as having average social skills. Although her global perception of Mike's social skills was average, she rated him as having fewer skills in the area of communication. For example, she rated him as "seldom" taking turns in or making eye contact during conversations.

Mrs. Stewart also appears to view Mike as having several maladaptive behaviors. For example, she noted that he often acts without thinking, is easily distracted, and becomes upset when his routine is changed.

At school, Mike's teachers view him as having typical social skills and few problem behaviors. One of Mike's teachers sees a need for him to assert himself more. Although Mike has generally typical social skills at school, he does not appear to have many friends and has difficulty with verbal comprehension.

Three teacher reports from December of DATE all describe Mike as having "excellent" or "average" relationships with his peers and adults. He is consistently described as "respectful" and having a positive attitude toward school.

Mrs. Hass said that Mike has one friend at school. She believes that Mike often pretends he comprehends things and will "talk around" things he does not understand. She thinks he needs things broken down into parts or steps for him to comprehend.

Both Mrs. Hass and Mr. Lopez, Mike's Life Science teacher, completed the teacher versions of the SSIS Rating Scale. Both Mrs. Hass and Mr. Lopez view Mike as having average social skills and average levels of maladaptive behaviors. Although Mr. Lopez views Mike's social skills as generally average, his ratings suggest that Mike may have fewer skills in the area of assertion than is typical. For example, Mr. Lopez said that Mike "never" "questions rules that may be unfair" and "seldom" "stands up for himself when treated unfairly."

What is the most appropriate educational diagnosis or special education classification for Mike?

At different times, Mike has been diagnosed as having a specific learning disability and a speech and language impairment. In addition, autism has been considered but ruled out on at least three occasions. The information from this and past assessments does not seem to support these diagnoses as the most appropriate diagnoses.

For example, Mike does not have a discrepancy between his academic achievement and his intellectual ability. In fact, his achievement, as assessed by both his performance on standardized tests and in the classroom, is better than what might be predicted by his assessed intellectual ability. In addition, Mike does not have the kind of inconsistency in his cognitive abilities that would suggest a specific or narrow cognitive weakness often associated with learning disabilities.

There is strong evidence that Mike's oral communication and language skills are significantly below those of his peers. Although this fits the state and federal definition for a student with a speech and language impairment, it does not seem that this diagnosis alone captures Mike's pattern of strengths and limitations.

The State Education Code defines *autism* in the following way: "A pupil exhibits any combination of the following autistic-like behaviors, to include but not limited to: (1) an inability to use oral language for appropriate communication; (2) a history of extreme withdrawal or relating to people inappropriately and continued impairment in social interaction from infancy through early childhood; (3) an obsession to maintain sameness; (4) extreme preoccupation with objects or inappropriate use of objects or both; (5) extreme resistance to controls; (6) displays peculiar motoric mannerisms and motility patterns; (7) self-stimulating, ritualistic behavior."

Although Mike has difficulties with verbal communication, this does not seem to constitute an "inability to use oral language for appropriate communication." Mike also does not appear to have "extreme withdrawal," "extreme resistance to controls," "peculiar motoric mannerisms," or "self-stimulating behavior." Mrs. Stewart describes Mike has having difficulty when his routine changes, but this does not seem to rise to the level of an "obsession to maintain sameness." Although Mike has limited friendships and does not seem as socially independent as others do his age, he appears to have good basic social skills. Taken together, these suggest that autism is not an appropriate educational diagnosis for Mike.

State Education Code defines an *intellectual disability* as consisting of two main components. One is "significantly subaverage general intellectual functioning." There is not a precise definition of *subaverage* in the educational code although standard scores on standardized tests of intelligence that fall between 70 and 75 are typically accepted as meeting this criterion. As noted above, Mike has a consistent pattern of subaverage performance on assessments of his general intellectual ability. These assessments have involved different tests and taken place over several years.

The second component of the definition of intellectual disability is having significantly fewer adaptive behavior skills than typical for a person's age. Mrs. Stewart's responses to the *Vineland Adaptive Behavior Scale II* suggest that Mike is much less independent than his peers are. According to Mrs. Stewart, Mike is more dependent on routines and parent prompting than typical for a student his age. Although Mike seems more independent at school, the evidence suggests that outside of the formal demands of school, he needs more structure and support than typical for students his age.

Given his history and pattern of scores and performances, it seems an educational diagnosis of intellectual disability best captures Mike's pattern of strengths and limitations.

What changes, if any, does Mike need in his IEP for him to continue to make adequate progress toward district and state academic standards?
Mike appears to be making adequate progress toward his IEP goals. If he continues to fail the High School Exit Exam, the IEP Team should consider further accommodations or exemption from the exam. At this point, Mike's current goals and services seem appropriate to meet his academic needs.

At the same time, Mike needs to learn to be more independent and be prepared for post-secondary life. In addition to learning to use public transportation, Mike should consider enrolling in a vocational class through the Local Occupational Program (LOP). For example, the LOP has classes in Music Technology, which may fit his interests.

The IEP Team may also consider setting up a work internship with a special education program so that Mike can gain experience as a classroom aide.

Mike also reports very limited interaction with others outside the classroom. Given this, he may benefit from some kind of informal friendship group where students who need to learn social skills meet to practice social skills in an informal setting with adult supervision.

Mike clearly does best with structure. Given this, it will be important for him to learn organizational skills such as using a calendar and keeping a to-do list that will allow him to begin to plan and structure his own time and tasks.

What changes, if any, are needed in Mike's Transition Plan for him to achieve his post-secondary goals?

Mike's current Individual Transition Plan includes activities such as completing a "pre-employment training" class, updating his resume, researching employment opportunities, developing self-advocacy skills, and developing a budget for living expenses. These seem appropriate although it would be helpful to break down in more detail the specific self-advocacy skills needed. This may be especially important given that one of Mike's teachers views him as having fewer assertion skills than typical for his age.

As discussed above, the IEP Team should also consider having Mike enroll in an LOP class of his choice and doing a work internship as a classroom aide. It may also be useful to have Mike visit local community colleges to explore their course offerings, programs, and admission processes. In addition to these activities, the IEP Team should consider connecting Mike to the Department of Rehabilitation for post-secondary services.

Example 2: Elementary Student, Initial Evaluation
Assessing for Specific Learning Disability Using RTI

This report is written at an 11.5 Flesch Kincaid grade level with 18% passive sentences.

Student: Max Wilson
Gender: Male
Age: 12.2
Grade: 5th

School: Ideal Elementary
Primary Language: English
Current Placement: Gen Ed

Reason for Referral: Max has attended Ideal Elementary School in Current Unified School District (CUSD) for 8 months. This school year Max received interventions to increase his reading fluency and writing skills. With this intensive support, Max's overall growth in language arts has been steady. However, he is at risk for retention because he is not meeting the district's fifth-grade literacy promotion standard. He was referred for a psychoeducational evaluation by the Students Success Team (SST) due to concerns with his academic progress in reading and written language. During interviews with Max's mother, she also noted significant environmental issues, including poor attendance due to multiple home and school changes, which she believes have negatively impacted Max's academic and emotional development. The focus of this evaluation is to determine Max's eligibility and need for special education services. The following questions were addressed as part of this evaluation:

- How do previous schooling, environmental factors, and health issues impact Max's current academic achievement?
- What are Max's current academic skills in reading, written language, and math?
- What is Max's general range of cognitive functioning and what are his cognitive processing strengths and weaknesses?
- How do Max's behavior and social emotional strengths and challenges affect his academic achievement?
- Is Max eligible for, and does he need, Special Education services to make progress in the general education curriculum?

Evaluation Procedures: The following evaluation procedures and assessment tools were used to gather information to answer the evaluation questions listed above.

Review of Records:

Cumulative School Records	DATE
Open Court Assessment Data	DATE
Classroom Work Samples	DATE

Interviews:

    Max Wilson, Student   DATE

    Ms. Wilson, Mother   DATE

    Mr. Lewis, 5th-Grade Teacher   DATE

    Ms. Intervention, Resource Specialist Program Teacher   DATE

Observations:

    Small-Group Guided Reading   DATE

    Whole-Class Direct Math Instruction   DATE

Standardized Assessments:

    Comprehensive Test of Phonological Processing (CTOPP)   DATE

    Behavior Assessment System for Children (BASC-3),

    Teacher Rating Scale (TRS)   DATE

Evaluation Questions and Answers: Throughout the assessment, Max was cooperative and willing to participate. Max appeared very comfortable throughout all of the testing and interview meetings. He put forth effort in all tasks and showed persistence even as tasks became more difficult. His levels of attention and concentration were all appropriate for his age. It is felt that the results of this evaluation provide a valid assessment of Max's current abilities and educational needs. The evaluation questions are used below as headings to organize this report. After each question, the answer is given in bold italics. The information used to come to these conclusions is presented below the answer.

How do previous schooling, environmental factors, and health issues impact Max's current academic achievement?

Max has a significant history of school changes and poor attendance. Due to this, it is clear that Max has received inconsistent instruction. Literacy interventions were implemented and modified over a 3-month period to evaluate Max's response to the intensive instruction in reading and written language. Max also has a history of demonstrating anxious behaviors related to home issues. He has received mental health services, and since his family life has stabilized his anxiety symptoms have significantly decreased. Max is in overall good health and his current school attendance is good.

Max is 12 years old and currently enrolled in fifth grade at Ideal Elementary School. Max has a history of multiple school and district changes and his academic records are incomplete. Based on a review of available school records, Max attended Kindergarten through the second trimester of second grade at Super Elementary School in Quality Unified School District. Max had poor attendance in Kindergarten and his initial year in first grade. He was retained in first grade, though his attendance remained poor. Max was provided interventions at Super Elementary, including small-group instruction, summer school, and at-risk Resource Specialist Program (RSP) services. Information regarding Max's response to these interventions was not in his school records. Assessing Max for Special Education services was mentioned in Student Success Team (SST) notes, though according to his mother an evaluation was not conducted.

Max transferred to Major Elementary within Another Unified School District to complete second grade. He was involved in a summer reading clinic and then attended third grade. An SST meeting was held to discuss Max's progress, and according to his mother an assessment for Special Education services was conducted. Ms. Wilson stated that Max was found to have "perceptual problems" but that he did not qualify for Special Education services. The report was not available to review for this evaluation.

Within the SST records, it also stated that there were concerns with issues of Tourette's and obsessive compulsive disorder. Ms. Wilson stated that Max has received mental health services for the past two years due to family issues of separation, spousal abuse, and homelessness. She stated that he used to demonstrate significant signs of anxiety, though was never diagnosed with the above disorders and it is unclear why they are mentioned in his school files. Now that Max's home life has stabilized, his mother reports that his anxiety issues have been minimized.

Max began attending school within the Current Unified School District (CUSD) in March of DATE. He enrolled as a fourth-grader at Hope School, a school exclusively for students who are homeless. In September of DATE, Max transferred to Ideal Elementary School to begin fifth grade. Since enrolling at Ideal, Max has had excellent attendance.

As part of this evaluation, a health assessment was completed on DATE. According to the nurse's report, Max's vision is 20/20 in both eyes. He passed the hearing screening at 25 decibels. Max is in the 60th percentile for his height and the 97th percentile for his weight. His immunizations are all current. He met all early developmental milestones within normal limits and has had no major illnesses or injuries. He is currently in good health.

What are Max's current academic skills in the areas of reading, written language, and math?

Max's current academic achievement was assessed through review of records, observations, teacher reports, interviews, and curriculum-based assessments. Although Max's academic skills in all areas have grown this school year, he continues to perform significantly below grade-level standards in reading and written language. Max's weakly developed phonics skills negatively impact his reading decoding, reading fluency, comprehension, and spelling.

Reading: Max's reading skills have improved since enrolling at Ideal Elementary. According to Mr. Lewis, Max has good oral comprehension of the Open Court stories when they are read aloud in class. He struggles with reading fluency and decoding. Mr. Lewis reported that Max's reading fluency is affected by his need to stop and decode words. When decoding multi-syllable words, Max often gets the first syllable and then guesses at the rest. Max's literal comprehension skills are strong, though he has difficulty with inferences when he cannot fluently read the text. He needs to be reminded to use reading comprehension strategies to support his understanding.

Max has recently passed the CUSD Mid-Third-Grade Reading Benchmark. Reading benchmarks are a CUSD-constructed measure of students' decoding and comprehension mastery. Students are given a benchmark assessment when they have demonstrated the skills to successfully pass the test at a given level. Max has passed four benchmarks since enrolling at Ideal, including the End of Second Grade and the Middle of Third-Grade Fiction and Nonfiction benchmarks.

In October, Max's average reading fluency was assessed at 39 words correct per minute. The goal level for a fifth-grader would be 90–120 words per minute. As part of the general education language arts program, Max worked with his teacher in small groups three times per week for 20 minutes on increasing fluency skills, decoding skills, and comprehension strategies. In November, Max's fluency was retested at 42 words per minute. Due to limited progress, a more intensive intervention was implemented. Max began working with the Resource Specialist Program (RSP) teacher two times per week in a small group for 30 minutes. Text rereading and sight-word memorization strategies were used to increase Max's reading fluency. A goal was set for Max to increase his fluency by 1.5 words per week. After 12 weeks, Max's fluency had increased to 51 words per minute. At that time, Max's intervention was increased to three times a week with the RSP teacher. Max's fluency 12 weeks after the increased level of intervention was 68.5 words read correctly per minute. With this level of intensive intervention Max was able to increase his fluency by 17.5 words in a 12-week period. He was able to meet his goal of increasing his reading fluency by 1.5 words per week, though he required a consistent and intensive level of support to be successful.

Written Language: Mr. Lewis reports that Max has good ideas, though he tends to write his thoughts into one paragraph. He uses many incomplete sentences and needs support editing for beginning capitalization and ending punctuation. When unsure of correct spelling, Max attempts to use phonetic rules though his spelling of sounds demonstrates weak phonetic knowledge. For example, in a writing sample Max spelled *roller skating* as "rodsating," *friend* as "frenid," and *weekend* as "wacand."

Max scored an average of 1 on a 4-point rubric on the first two Open Court Unit writing assessments. A score of 3 demonstrates proficient skills. In January, Mr. Lewis began working with Max in a small group two times per week on editing for spelling, punctuation, and sentence structure. Max has increased his average Open Court writing assessment score on Units 4, 5, and 6 to a 1.8 on the 4-point rubric.

Math: Math is Max's academic strength. He has made significant progress this school year. Max entered fifth grade with inconsistent multiplication skills. He is currently advanced proficient on addition, subtraction, multiplication, and division facts tests. He is able to consistently score at a 97% level or better within 5 minutes on these tests. Max's performance on the first and second trimester math assessment was in the proficient range. He consistently meets grade-level standards in computing problems and accessing and solving word problems.

How do Max's cognitive processing strengths or weaknesses impact his academic achievement?

Max's cognitive abilities were assessed through observations, teacher interviews, parent interviews, and standardized assessment. His overall general cognitive ability is estimated to be in the average range. Based on standardized assessments, classroom observations, and teachers' reports, Max demonstrates a significant weakness in the area of phonological awareness. Max's weaknesses in phonological processing impact his overall literacy skills.

Max demonstrates many behaviors and skills consistent with solidly average cognitive ability. Max is proficient with grade-level math computation and applied problems. Max demonstrates leadership qualities in nonacademic areas and has well-developed social skills with peers and adults. He resolves conflict thoughtfully and logically. Max is able to engage in age-level conversations with peers and adults. He gives appropriate and sequential explanations and is able to describe nonacademic interests and experiences with detail. He shows creativity in stories told and questions asked. Max has strong listening comprehension skills. He remembers information and facts, from stories read to the class, as well as movies and television programs he has watched at home. Max also demonstrates a clever sense of humor. He understands and uses jokes, riddles, and humor that many of his peers do not yet completely grasp.

Max's phonological awareness was assessed because of the weak phonetic skills he demonstrates in the classroom. The Comprehensive Test of Phonological Processing (CTOPP) is a standardized measure designed to assess phonological awareness, phonological memory, and rapid naming. These three types of phonological processing are important skills for learning how to read and write.

The Phonological Awareness Composite Score is a measure of an individual's phonological awareness and understanding of the sounds in oral language. Good phonological awareness is associated with good decoding and reading skills. Max's performance on this measure was in the significantly below-average range. The Phonological Memory Composite is a measure of an individual's ability to work with phonological information. The Rapid Naming Composite Score is a measure of retrieval speed of phonological information from long-term or permanent memory. Max's performance on both of these measures was solidly within the average range. There is a significant discrepancy between Max's performance on the Phonological Awareness Composite and his performances on the Phonological Memory and Rapid Naming Composites, suggesting that Phonological Awareness is a significant area of weakness. Max's weakness in phonological awareness is also evident in his classwork. Max demonstrates slow fluency when reading due to his difficulty decoding unfamiliar words. He also has difficulty utilizing phonetic skills when encoding, or spelling unknown words.

How do Max's behavior and social-emotional strengths and challenges affect his academic achievement?

Max is a responsible and motivated student, which positively impacts his academic achievement. He has worked hard this school year and made significant academic growth.

During interviews, Ms. Wilson reported a history of significant anxiety for Max. Because of this history, an evaluation of Max's current emotional status was conducted. The *Behavior Assessment System for Children–3* (BASC-3), a multidimensional system used to evaluate the behavior and self-perceptions of children and young adults aged 2 through 25 years, was used to aide in assessing Max's behavior and emotional status at school. Max's teacher completed the Teacher Rating Scale. Several attempts were made, though Max's mother did not return the Parent Rating Scale. However, Ms. Wilson did provide information about Max's behavior and social and emotional development through interviews.

The Teacher Rating Scale is a comprehensive measure of a child's adaptive and problem behaviors in a school setting. BASC-3 scores within the clinically significant range suggest a student has many symptoms or problem behaviors and is having significant difficulties in everyday life. Scores in the at-risk range may identify a potential problem. Scores in the typical range suggest that Max's behavior is similar to his peers and that he is functioning normally in the school environment. According to Mr. Lewis's ratings of Max's behavior, all scores fell in normal limits, suggesting he observes no emotional issues or behaviors in class that negatively impact Max's achievement. Areas in which he noted that Max had well-developed skills were Adaptability, Social Skills, Leadership, Study Skills, and Functional Communication.

During interviews, Mr. Lewis has also stated that Max is a responsible student. He arrives at school on time and ready to learn. Max is a hard worker and completes class and homework assignments. He begins and completes work in a timely manner and exhibits motivation to learn. Max is very respectful to peers and adults and is well liked by all. He follows school and classroom rules, though he can be talkative due to his social nature.

Is Max eligible for, and does he need, Special Education services to make progress in the general education curriculum?

Max is eligible for services as a student demonstrating a specific learning disability (SLD). He has been provided intensive reading interventions, which he continues to need to make continued academic growth toward grade-level standards. Max also demonstrates significant weaknesses in phonological awareness. He needs Special Education services to make progress toward grade-level curriculum.

Max is a 12-year-old boy currently enrolled in the fifth grade at Ideal Elementary School. This assessment was completed to evaluate Max's current eligibility and need for further Special Education services. Based on interviews, observations, and testing, Max demonstrates overall cognitive ability within the average range. Max's academic achievement in basic reading skills and written language is significantly below grade-level standards. He also demonstrates significant weaknesses in phonological awareness. With an intensive level of intervention in the areas of reading fluency and writing, Max has demonstrated academic growth, though the level of support needed cannot be provided in the general education classroom. He is eligible for Special Education services as a student demonstrating a specific learning disability (SLD), which negatively impacts his academic achievement. An Individualized Education Program (IEP) meeting will convene to review these assessment results. Decisions regarding both eligibility and services will be made by the IEP team.

The following recommendations should be reviewed by the IEP team:

- Max has successfully transitioned to his new school this year. He will transfer to a middle school for sixth grade this fall. To support a smooth transition and continued academic and social success, the counselor will work with Max's mother on choosing an appropriate middle school. The counselor will also contact Max's middle school counselor to share successful supports for Max.
- Max has demonstrated excellent leadership skills and he is well liked by other students. Encouraging Max to join clubs and/or sports teams in middle school will help to continue his success with peer relationships.
- Max has weak phonetic skills. Based on the reading assessment he needs continued instruction and practice with decoding irregular vowels and diphthongs.
- Max can currently read and spell the first 200 sight-words in the Frye sight-word list. The Frye list contains the most common words in print. Continued practice with the next 200 words will improve his fluency and accuracy in both reading and writing.

Respectfully Submitted,
School Psychologist

Example 3: High School Student, Reevaluation
Assessing for an Emotional Disturbance

This report is written at an 11.0 Flesch Kincaid grade level with 12% passive sentences.

Name: Darion Brady
Chronological Age: 15-3

Reason for Referral and Assessment Questions:
This is Darion's second psychoeducational evaluation. He was last evaluated in February of DATE. The focus of that evaluation was on whether Darion qualified for special education services as a student with an attention-deficit/hyperactivity disorder (ADHD) or a specific learning disability. The evaluation concluded that Darion did not meet the criteria for either ADHD or a learning disability. Darion failed three classes last year and is currently failing two more classes. He continues to struggle to complete work and attend school regularly. His parents also report five suicide attempts since March of DATE and both his parents and school personnel are concerned about his ability to cope with the demands of a comprehensive high school.

The current assessment is being conducted to answer the following questions:

1. What are Darion's present levels of academic, cognitive, social, and emotional development?
2. Does Darion have an emotional disturbance as defined by federal and state regulations?
3. What supports are necessary to help Darion make adequate progress toward state and district academic standards? Does he need special education services in order to meet these expectations?

Assessment Procedures:
1. Review of school records, including a Multidisciplinary Assessment Team Report written in February of DATE.
2. Phone interview with Darion's psychotherapist, Dr. Busse, on 1/25/DATE.
3. Darion was interviewed on 1/12/DATE. He also completed the *Behavior Assessment System for Children, Third Edition, Self-Report of Personality* on the same date. He was interviewed again on 2/15/DATE.
4. Mr. and Mrs. Brady were interviewed on 1/17/DATE. They also completed the *Behavior Assessment System for Children III Parent Rating Scales* on 2/8/DATE.

5. Darion's Language Arts and World History teachers completed the *Behavior Assessment System for Children III Teacher Rating Scales* on 1/12 and 1/17/DATE.

Background Information and Record Review:
Darion's background information was gathered from the Multidisciplinary Assessment Team Report written in February of DATE, a *Structured Developmental History* completed by Mrs. Brady, and an interview with Mr. and Mrs. Brady on 1/17/DATE.

Darion lives at home with his adoptive parents and his 14-year-old adopted sister. Mrs. Brady is an elementary school teacher and Mr. Brady works as a produce manager for Big Box Grocery Stores.

Darion was adopted at birth. According to Mrs. Brady, he and his biological mother were healthy at his birth. Mrs. Brady does not recall Darion's early developmental milestones but does not remember having any concerns about his development, including eating, sleeping, learning to walk, or learning to talk. Darion's vision and hearing are normal and he is currently in good physical health.

Mr. and Mrs. Brady describe Darion as "normal" until seventh grade. In seventh and eighth grades, they viewed him as "happy" but he began to have difficulty completing schoolwork. In the summer after eighth grade, he began to see a private psychotherapist to help the family "set limits." Mr. and Mrs. Brady report that this therapist thought that Darion had a "borderline personality disorder."

In ninth grade, Darion began to report that he did not want to go to school because of being bullied. Darion and his parents reported these incidents to the school counselor, but she was unable to identify the perpetrators or gather sufficient information from Darion to intervene.

Darion's parents referred him to the school for an evaluation toward the end of his first semester in ninth grade because of their concerns he might have attention-deficit/ hyperactivity disorder (ADHD) or a specific learning disability. This evaluation concluded that Darion had average cognitive and academic skills and did not have ADHD or a learning disability. Aside from attention, this evaluation did not focus on Darion's social and emotional functioning.

In March of his ninth-grade year, Darion attempted to strangle himself by wrapping a towel around his neck. He was hospitalized for three days at College Hospital, a local psychiatric facility. Following this, Darion began to see another psychotherapist,

Dr. Busse. In the fall of his 11th-grade year, Darion made three more suicide attempts over the course of about two months. These attempts included taking multiple doses of the medication Abilify and cutting his arm. Each time, he was taken to the emergency room and released. Most recently, Darion made a fifth suicide attempt following an argument with his mother about homework. He was hospitalized for three days at State University Medical Center. According to his parents, Darion has been referred to a day-treatment program at State University. As of the time of this report, Darion had not yet started attending the program.

Currently, Darion sees Dr. Busse weekly. During a phone interview on 1/25/DATE, Dr. Busse described Darion as someone who becomes "stuck" in negative perceptions. He said that Darion is struggling with the issue of his adoption and feels disconnected from his adoptive parents. Dr. Busse also stated that although borderline personality disorder is a possible diagnosis, he believes that it is more likely that Darion has a mood disorder such as major depression or dysthymic disorder.

Darion also sees a psychiatrist, Dr. Le, who manages his medications. When this evaluation began, Darion was taking Abilify and Welbutrin. Abilify is used to treat a variety of psychiatric conditions, including psychosis, the manic symptoms of bipolar disorder, and depression when the symptoms are not controlled by an antidepressant medication alone. Welbutrin is an antidepressant. At the time of his second interview and following another suicide attempt and hospitalization, Darion stopped taking Abilify and Welbutrin and began taking Zoloft. Zoloft is in a class of antidepressant medications called *selective serotonin reuptake inhibitors* (SSRIs).

Darion transferred from Local High School to Wiley High School at the end of January DATE. During his first semester at Local High School, he had eight excused absences. He has missed seven days since enrolling at Wiley High School on 1/30/DATE. His parents report that he often complains of not feeling well and has sometimes refused to go to school.

Assessment Results:

What are Darion's present levels of academic, cognitive, social, and emotional development?

> *Although Darion has average cognitive ability and academic skills, he failed three classes last year and is failing two classes this semester. He has completed 50 of 180 credits required for high school graduation with a 2.0 GPA.*

In January of DATE, Darion had completed 50 of the 180 credits needed for high school graduation. His high school grade point average was 2.0 and he failed three classes his ninth grade year, which leaves him 15 credits behind what would normally be expected after completing ninth grade. Darion has not yet taken the High School Exit Exam.

At the end of the second quarter of the fall semester, Darion had A's in Vocal Ensemble and Athletics. He had C's in World History and Language Arts and F's in Algebra and Biology. Both low test scores and missing or incomplete assignments are noted in the teacher comments on his report card for the classes he is failing. In Vocal Ensemble, the teacher noted he was a "pleasure to have in class."

In February of DATE, Darion was given both the *Woodcock Johnson IV Tests of Achievement* (WJ IV ACH) and the *Woodcock Johnson IV Tests of Cognitive Ability* (WJ IV COG). On the WJ IV COG, Darion's general intellectual ability was average (GIA standard score range of 94 to 112). He had significant personal strengths in auditory processing and short-term memory, including working memory. Academically, Darion's performance on the WJ IV ACH in reading, written language, and math were all in the average range.

> *Darion has tried to commit suicide five times in the last year. He has friends and participates in several extracurricular activities but views himself as having many more symptoms of depression than is typical for adolescents his age.*

When Darion was interviewed on 1/12/DATE, he was cooperative, open, and answered questions willingly. Although he was cooperative, Darion's affect seemed subdued and he expressed a limited range of emotions.

Darion said he enjoyed soccer and singing in the school vocal ensemble. He also enjoys surfing, snowboarding, taking karate lessons, and riding his scooter competitively. He reported that he has three friends at school and hangs out with four or five friends on the weekend. Although Darion has friends, he complained that he feels stressed about being bullied at school. When asked to describe the bullying, Darion said that people at school make fun of him or make mean comments when he walks by.

Darion described four incidents where he attempted to take his own life that had occurred up to the time of this first interview. These included cutting his arm, trying to strangle himself, taking pills, and trying to hang himself. When asked what led to these attempts, Darion said he did not like his life and was tired of being bullied and not getting along with his parents.

Darion said he felt sad about 70% of the time and anxious about 40% of the time. He also has problems sleeping because his mind is racing. When asked to rate how things were going in his life on a scale of 1 to 10 (1 = low and 10 = high) Darion said things were a 5 or 6, which was a little better than a month ago when he would have given himself a 4. He said that he was getting along better with his friends and his parents and had recently been "sponsored" for riding his scooter. As noted above, Darion was taking two medications, Abilify, and one other medication he could not remember. He did not think the Abilify helped but thought the second medication might be helping a little.

Following this interview, Darion completed the *Behavior Assessment System for Children, Third Edition, Self-Report of Personality* (BASC-3 SRP). The BASC-3 SRP asks students to respond to a series of questions and statements as "true" or "false" on a four-point scale ranging from "never" to "almost always." The Clinical scales on the BASC-3 SRP provide an assessment of self-perceived social and emotional problems while the Adaptive scales evaluate positive coping and social skills.

Darion's responses to the BASC-3 SRP suggest that he sees himself as having typical interpersonal relations and a feeling of self-reliance. For example, he responded "almost always" to questions like "I am dependable," "My friends come to me for help," and "I am liked by others."

His responses also suggest he views himself as having many more symptoms of depression than other adolescents (*t*-score of 82) have. Darion responded "true" or "almost always" to 9 of the 12 questions on the BASC-3 SRP depression scale. For example, he said he "almost always" felt depressed and that life was getting worse and worse. He responded "true" to statements like "Nothing is fun anymore" and "I just don't care anymore."

Darion also has more feelings of inadequacy (*t*-score of 70) and lower self-esteem (*t*-score of 35) than is typical for students his age. Difficulties in these areas are often associated with depression and further suggest that depression is a significant concern.

Darion also views himself as having many more behaviors than other students that might be considered odd or unusual. On the BASC-3 SRP, the Atypicality scale (*t*-score of 99) measures these behaviors. Darion responded "almost always," "often," or "true" to 7 of the 9 questions on the Atypicality scale. This included responding, "almost always" to questions like "I hear voices in my head that no one else can hear," "I hear things that others cannot hear," and "Even when I am alone, I feel like someone is watching me."

When interviewed on 2/15/DATE, Darion had recently been hospitalized again for a fifth suicide attempt following a transfer to Wiley High School from Local High.

He said that things were going pretty well at school but not very well at home. Darion said he had not had any thoughts of suicide since being released about a week before the interview. When asked how often he feels sad or depressed, Darion said he now felt sad about 40% of the time (compared to 70% on 1/1). He also said he was not getting as mad as before and that his new medication (Zoloft) seemed to be helping.

Darion was also asked about his reports on the BASC-3 SRP of hearing voices. He said that he sometimes would hear his biological mother call his name at night. He reported that he heard voices before when he felt "scared and depressed" but no longer heard voices. Darion also said he still worried about losing his friends and being alone but no longer worried about "every little thing." When asked to account for these changes, Darion said he had learned some new coping skills while in the hospital and that he was now taking an antidepressant, Zoloft, rather than Abilify. He said that the Zoloft seemed to help him "not get as mad."

> *Darion's parents view him as having friends and average social skills but many more symptoms of depression than typical. They describe him as less motivated toward school and his extracurricular activities such as choir and soccer. Most of his five suicide attempts have followed arguments with his parents over mundane things such as homework or phone privileges.*

In an interview on 1/17/DATE, Mr. and Mrs. Brady said they believed that Darion was a "normal" student until seventh grade, when he began to have problems completing his schoolwork. In ninth grade he began to complain of being bullied at school and in March of ninth grade, he made the first of five suicide attempts. These attempts often followed arguments between Darion and his parents and attempts on their part to discipline him. For example, Darion's first suicide attempt followed his father taking his phone away. The most recent attempt followed an argument with his mother about homework and his refusal to go to school.

Mr. and Mrs. Brady describe Darion as not liking crowds but also not liking to be alone. He interacts with friends on a regular basis and has a girlfriend who attends Wiley High School. Darion has also been involved in several activities, including soccer, surfing, choir, and riding his scooter. They note that in the last few months he has withdrawn from soccer and choir and says he does not want to go to school.

Darion's parents also completed the *Behavior Assessment System for Children–3 Parent Rating Scales* (BASC-3 PRS). The BASC-3 PRS is designed to assess parents' perceptions of their children's pro-social or adaptive skills, externalizing problems (hyperactivity, aggression, problems of conduct), and internalizing problems (anxiety, depression, somatization).

Both Mr. and Mrs. Brady view Darion as having average social skills, functional communication, and adaptability (adjusting to changes in routine, etc.), but they also view him as having many more symptoms of depression than his peers do (*t*-scores of 85 and 110*)*. Both responded "often" or "almost always" to questions such as "is negative about things," "says, 'I hate myself,'" and "says, 'I want to die' or 'I wish I were dead.'" Darion's parents also view him as having more symptoms of anxiety than typical, although this appears to be a less severe problem than depression.

> *Two of Darion's teachers completed the Behavior Assessment System for Children–3 Teacher Rating Scales. Neither sees him as having significant problems but at the same time both view him as having difficulty interacting positively with other students.*

Two of Darion's teachers at Local High School completed the *Behavior Assessment System for Children–3 Teacher Rating Scales* (BASC-3 TRS). Like the BASC-3 SRP and BASC-3 PRS, the BASC-3 TRS assesses perceptions of both problem behaviors and adaptive skills. Neither Darion's Science teacher nor his Economics teacher view him as having significant problems with acting out, depression, or anxiety, but both view him as having fewer social skills than typical. Specifically, they appear to see him as having difficulty interacting positively with others. For example, both teachers state that Darion "never" "offers to help other adolescents," "compliments others," or "congratulates others when good things happen to them."

Does Darion have an emotional disturbance as defined by federal and state regulations?

According to state and federal regulations, to meet Special Education eligibility as a student with an emotional disturbance, a student must have one of the following conditions:

1. An inability to learn that cannot be explained by intellectual, sensory, or health factors.
2. An inability to build or maintain satisfactory interpersonal relationships with peers and teachers.

3. Inappropriate types of behavior or feelings under normal circumstances.
4. A general pervasive mood of unhappiness or depression.
5. A tendency to develop physical symptoms or fears associated with personal or school problems.

If present, these conditions must (a) have existed for a long time, (b) be present to a marked degree, and (c) have a significant negative impact on educational performance.

Darion appears to meet these criteria. Of these conditions, there is strong evidence that Darion has "a general pervasive mood of unhappiness." Darion has made five suicide attempts in the last year and been hospitalized twice. In addition, he is currently being treated with antidepressant medication. His responses to the BASC-3 SRP suggest that he has many more symptoms of depression than are typical. Although he views himself as improved over the course of the evaluation, Darion still says he is sad 40% of the time. Darion's parents also view him as having many symptoms of depression. His suicide attempts have followed arguments with his parents over ordinary issues such as completing homework and phone privileges. This suggests that Darion is struggling to adequately regulate his emotions and cope appropriately.

Darion's symptoms of depression, including attempts at suicide, have been present for almost a year. During that time, he has failed three classes and is currently failing two more. If he fails two of his current classes, Darion will be 25 credits behind what is expected of an 11th-grade student. This is in spite of average cognitive abilities and academic skills.

What supports are necessary to help Darion make adequate progress toward state and district academic standards? Does he need special education services in order to meet these expectations?
At this point, it appears that Darion will need the monitoring and support provided by a special education program. At the same time, given his cognitive and academic strengths, every effort should be made to keep him in general education classes where he can benefit from the general education curriculum. The IEP team should consider goals in the areas of attendance, work completion, and emotional self-regulation. In order to accomplish goals in these areas, the IEP team might consider assigning Darion a special education case carrier who can monitor his progress in his general education classes and respond quickly to absences. The case carrier can also be a liaison between school and Darion's treatment providers, such as Dr. Busse.

Darion also appears to have significant signs of depression. He should be strongly encouraged to continue his current treatment, including participation in the recommended State University day-treatment program. In addition, the school staff should support Darion's involvement in extracurricular activities such as choir and athletics.

School-based individual or group counseling for Darion can also help him learn self-regulatory skills such as identifying and monitoring his emotions. For example, Darion could keep a mood diary that could be reviewed regularly with his case carrier or counselor (at first this might be done daily but could be reduced to weekly as Darion develops greater mindfulness and control of his emotions). Darion's case carrier, perhaps with the assistance of the School Counselor or School Psychologist, should also develop a menu of appropriate ways Darion can cope if he feels depressed or distressed. Given the link between Darion's suicide attempts and his reports of being bullied, the school counselor or school administrator should closely investigate and, if needed, intervene in any incidents of Darion being bullied.

Appendix II

Example 4: Elementary Student, Initial Evaluation
Assessing for Learning Disability and Other Health Impairment

This report is written at an 11.7 Flesch Kincaid grade level with 17% passive sentences.

Student: April Campbell   **School:** Smith Primary Academy
Gender: Female   **Primary Language:** English
Age: 6.0   **Current Placement:** General Education
Grade: K

Reason for Referral: April is a Kindergarten student enrolled in Current Unified School District (CUSD) at Smith Primary Academy. April was diagnosed with neurofibromatosis (NF1), a neurocutaneous genetic syndrome, at the age of 5 months. The severity of NF1 varies greatly and can present with different physical signs and complications for each person. Currently, April's medical needs are monitored through a neurologist and orthopedist at Children's Hospital. She wears a brace to support and protect her left leg and has some physical limitations, including no jumping or pounding activities to protect her leg from physical impact.

For the 20XX school year, April attended a CUSD pre-Kindergarten program at Brookside Elementary School. She made slow academic progress and had difficulty retaining much of the academic information she learned. April has been receiving 90 minutes of weekly literacy intervention since the beginning of October. April's parents and current Kindergarten teacher were concerned with possible learning delays, which are often associated with NF1. April's mother, Mrs. Campbell, requested a psychoeducational evaluation be conducted to evaluate April's eligibility and need for Special Education services. Due to April's medical history and current concerns with learning, the eligibilities of Specific Learning Disability and Other Health Impairment will be evaluated. This psychoeducational evaluation will answer the following questions:

- How does April's developmental, medical, and educational history affect her current academic achievement?
- What are April's current academic skills in the areas of reading, written language, and math?
- What are April's cognitive processing strengths and weaknesses?
- Does April qualify for and need Special Education services to make progress toward grade-level academic standards?

145

Assessment Procedures:

Review of Records:

Cumulative School Records	DATE
Classroom Work Samples	DATE
CUSD Criterion-Based Assessments	DATE

Interviews:

Teacher, Rose Patience	DATE
Student, April Campbell	DATE
Mother, Lisa Campbell	DATE

Observations:

Kindergarten Classroom: Whole-Group Language Arts Instruction	DATE
Kindergarten Classroom: Recess	DATE

Standardized Assessments:

Differential Ability Scales–2	DATE

Assessment Questions and Results: Throughout the direct assessment, April was cooperative and willing to participate. She easily engaged in conversation and readily smiled when provided positive feedback. At times, April would become off-task by asking when she could return to her classroom. However, she was easily redirected to task through verbal prompts and a promise that she would not miss her recess with her friends. The assessment questions addressed within this report are listed as headings below. After each question, the answer is provided in bold italics. The information and data used to answer the questions are also provided in the narrative following each question. Specific scores on standardized assessments are included on the last page of the report.

How does April's developmental, medical, and educational history affect her current academic achievement?

April is an active and engaged Kindergartener in Mrs. Patience's classroom. She has neurofibromatosis (NF1), a genetic neurological syndrome. Her mother noted that she currently has mild symptoms, which are monitored by a neurologist and orthopedist. April is currently in good health. April completed a pre-Kindergarten program last school year and has transitioned to Kindergarten at Smith Primary Academy. She is making academic progress, though her teacher has some concerns with her retention.

April's background history was gathered through a review of school records and an interview with her mother, Lisa Campbell. According to Mrs. Campbell, her pregnancy with April was healthy with no complications. April was born full term. Both Mrs. Campbell and April were healthy and released from the hospital after one day. April began seeing her pediatrician at two weeks of age for well-baby examinations. The family noted that April's right leg was developing at an odd angle and that she had multiple café-au-lait spots (small coffee-colored patches). According to April's mother, their pediatrician had similar concerns and April's development was closely monitored.

April met all early physical, social, and language developmental milestones. She was visually tracking, smiling, babbling, and beginning to sit up at 4 months. April was first seen by a neurologist and geneticist at the age of 5 months due to concerns with an increase in the number of café-au-lait spots. After further testing, April was diagnosed with neurofibromatosis (NF1). According to Mrs. Campbell, features of NF1 may include café-au-lait spots, neurofibromas (tumors on, under, or hanging off the skin), Lisch nodules (tiny, noncancerous tumors on the iris), freckling in the folds of the skin, abnormalities of the skeleton, such as the thinning or overgrowth of the bones in the arms or lower leg, and curvature of the spine (scoliosis). The severity of NF1 varies greatly and can present with different physical signs and complications for each person. Treatment for NF1 often includes removal of the neurofibromas for cosmetic purposes, treating the complications, and getting intervention for children with learning disabilities since approximately 50% of students with NF demonstrate learning disabilities. Children are usually followed by appropriate medical specialists to monitor and treat complications. April initially presented with multiple café-au-lait spots, a neurofibroma on her chin, Lisch nodules, freckling in the folds of her skin, and thinning in the bones in the right lower leg. She is currently followed by Dr. Stellar, a neurologist, and Dr. Femur, an orthopedic surgeon, at Children's Hospital.

Due to significant bone thinning, April broke her right leg at 10 months of age. It was casted until her initial surgery in December of DATE. In February of DATE, a second surgery was conducted and April began wearing a protective brace. April's physical and gross motor development has been typical, despite breaks and surgeries on her leg. In March of DATE, a neurofibroma was removed from April's chin. A second removal surgery was conducted in February of DATE. Mrs. Campbell noted that the neurofibromas cannot be permanently removed and multiple surgeries may be needed.

At the age of 12 months, April received 11 months of early intervention physical and occupational therapy services through Local Regional Center. Mrs. Campbell reported that they helped April learn to safely walk and play with her brace. At the age of 3, April participated in a play-based preschool program for 6 hours a week. She enrolled in a pre-Kindergarten (pre-K) program at Bookside Elementary School in September of DATE. April's mother noted that she made slow academic progress over the school year. According to her report card, April completed the school year mastering some beginning phonemic awareness skills such as rhyming and identifying beginning and ending word sounds. April was able to identify 10 uppercase- and 8 lowercase-letter names, 8-letter sounds, and 9 high-frequency sight-words. April passed the CUSD Beginning of Kindergarten reading benchmark, a measure of basic book concepts and comprehension of a picture story. She was considered an emergent writer and was meeting some pre-K math expectations.

April enrolled at Smith Primary Academy in September of DATE. She is in Mrs. Patience's Kindergarten classroom. On September, DATE, a Student Success Team (SST) meeting was held to discuss April's medical and safety needs and her transition to Kindergarten. April's mother was very concerned with April's retention of academic skills and how her NF1 symptoms might impact April's academic achievement and performance. Due to concerns with her retention of academic skills, a literacy intervention was put into place while an evaluation for Special Education services was conducted. April has received direct services from the Resource Specialist Program (RSP) three times per week for 30 minutes. She is working on letter names, letter sounds, and writing.

April currently wears a patella tendon brace to support and protect her leg and has some limitations, including no jumping or pounding activities to protect her leg from physical impact. A safety plan is in place and April, school administration, and playground staff have been made aware of her limitations. At school and home, April is encouraged to engage in alternative physical activity for bone growth. The nurse conducted an initial health screening on 10-19-DATE. April's vision was 20/30 in each eye and 20/20 when using both eyes. She passed the hearing screening at 25 dB. Besides issues related to NF1, April has been a healthy child and her immunizations are current.

What are April's current academic skills in the areas of reading, written language, and math?

April's current academic achievement was assessed through review of records, observations, teacher reports, interviews, classroom work samples, and criterion-based assessments. April had difficulty retaining many of the academic skills presented in her pre-Kindergarten classroom, though since September she has made steady progress in mastering beginning Kindergarten reading, writing, and math skills. April's work habits are developing. She sometimes needs adult encouragement to stay engaged in instruction, try new things, and put forth her best effort.

Language Arts: CUSD uses reading benchmarks to assess students' reading mastery. Reading benchmarks are given when the teacher believes the student has demonstrated the literacy skills to pass the reading assessment at a specific level. April passed the Beginning Kindergarten reading benchmark, a measure of basic book concepts and comprehension of a picture story during her year in pre-Kindergarten (pre-K). April completed her pre-K program with some letter-name and -sound knowledge, though she did not retain this information over the summer break. April's progress was slow in the beginning of the year, but Mrs. Patience recently noted that her rate of learning and retention has increased and that she is happy with April's progress. The graph below shows April's pre-reading skills progress since the end of pre-K.

	June DATE (pre-Kindergarten)	September DATE (Kindergarten)	October DATE (Kindergarten)
Uppercase Letter Names	10/26	6/26	19/26
Lowercase Letter Names	8/28	4/28	14/28
Letter Sounds	8/26	0/26	24/26
Sight-Words	7/10	0/10	7/10

At the end of October, April knew 33/54 letter names and 24/26 letter sounds, which is consistent with many students in her classroom. Mrs. Patience noted that April was also growing in her writing. She began the year only drawing dog pictures and writing the word "DOG." With encouragement from her teacher, she is expanding her writing through using her knowledge of letter sounds to spell unknown words. She is becoming more confident in her writing and beginning to stretch words out and use more sight-words. April is right-handed and uses a correct pencil grip. She braces the paper with her left hand when writing.

Math: Math is April's strongest subject. She completed pre-K partially proficient in number sense and beginning math concepts. Mrs. Patience noted that April learns new math concepts easily and is able to complete grade-level work with accuracy. She can identify numbers to 30 and has scored in the advanced proficient range on the first two math assessments.

Classroom Adaptive Skills: April's work habits in the classroom are improving. April needs support from adults to take academic risks. She will complete work that is given to her, though has needed encouragement from her teacher to expand her skills and try new things. April sometimes needs prompts from her teacher to refocus and do her best work during whole-group instruction and independent work. April can be fidgety in class, often playing with little pieces of paper she finds. She can also be very social and enjoys engaging in conversation with her classmates. She accepts teacher redirection and often gives her teacher a big, bright-eyed smile when she is prompted to get back to work.

April is an active participant in the classroom. She enjoys sharing her ideas and working with her classmates. Mrs. Patience noted that she is well liked by her peers and has made friends. April can be impulsive in the classroom and at recess, which can lead to rougher play than some of her classmates want to engage in. April reports that recess and lunchtime are her favorite school activities. During an observation of April during recess, she was actively running and playing a game of chase with other students. She had a big smile and laugh, and enjoyed being a leader in the game.

What are April's cognitive processing strengths and weaknesses?

April's cognitive abilities were assessed through observations, teacher interviews, parent interviews, and standardized assessment. April's overall cognitive ability is estimated to be in the average range. During testing, April demonstrated relative strengths and weaknesses, though her overall cognitive processing abilities were all within an average range.

The *Differential Ability Scales–2 (DAS-2)* is a standardized nationally normed, individually administered assessment battery designed to evaluate cognitive processing in students 2 years, 6 months through 17 years, 11 months of age. April was given the DAS-2 Early Years Core Subtests and selected Diagnostic Subtests. The General Cognitive Ability (GCA) is a global ability estimate calculated using the results of the three DAS-2 Cluster scores (Verbal, Nonverbal Reasoning, and Spatial). The GCA is considered the score that is most representative of general intellectual ability; however, April's performance on the three clusters was significantly different so it is more appropriate to interpret her performance within each of the specific cluster areas.

Cluster scores are estimates of overall functioning in broadly defined cognitive domains. The Verbal cluster is a measure of acquired or learned verbal concepts and knowledge. This cluster is comprised of the Verbal Comprehension and Naming Vocabulary subtests. April's performance on the Verbal cluster was in the above-average range. April demonstrated well-developed language comprehension on the Verbal Comprehension subtest. She was able to follow multistep directions and match stories to pictures. Her ability to identify common objects in the Naming Vocabulary subtest was in the above-average range. She demonstrated a strong vocabulary, even when she was unable to identify the picture. For example, when asked for the word *eruption*, April stated, "the volcano is ready to blow with hot lava."

The Nonverbal Reasoning Ability cluster is a measure of nonverbal mental processing, inductive reasoning, and visual processing. The Matrixes and Picture Similarities subtests are included in this cluster. April's performance on the Non-Verbal Reasoning cluster was in the average range. April was able to visually separate patterns or puzzles into their components, draw conclusions, and solve them using her knowledge base. April did especially well on the Picture Similarities subtest where she was asked to match pictures with a common element or concept.

The Spatial Ability cluster is a measure of complex visual-spatial processing. Copying, a measure of visual perceptual matching and fine-motor coordination in copying line drawings, and Pattern Construction, a measure of spatial visualization and orientation in copying block patterns, are the subtests included in this cluster. Both of these subtests involve motor planning, as the student must recreate designs either through drawing or using blocks. April's performance on this cluster was in the below-average range, though her performances on the two subtests that comprise this cluster were significantly different. Specifically, April's performance on the Pattern Construction subtest was in the average range. She worked slowly, though accurately, and at one point during this timed test, looked up, smiled, and asked, "Why are we doing this?" April's performance on the Copying subtest was in the below-average range, though this needs to be interpreted with caution. April was very concerned about missing her recess and knew this was her last task before we were finished. She seemed to rush through many of the drawings, which affected her score. When asked to slow down and recopy the drawings, April's ability greatly improved. She used proper pencil grip and braced the paper when drawing. She knew when she made a mistake and asked to redo two of her drawings. In the classroom, April's penmanship is best when she is given lined paper for boundaries and encouraged to do her best work. Her letter formation has continued to improve since the beginning of the school year. April's lower performance on this subtest appears to be due to her rushed efforts, not a delay in fine-motor development or visual spatial matching.

Diagnostic subtests of the DAS-2 were used to further evaluate April's cognitive processing skills. The Phonological Processing subtest of the Differential Ability Scales (DAS-2) is a measure of the knowledge of sound structure of the English language and the ability to manipulate sound. Phonological awareness helps children learn how letters and sounds go together in written language, which supports learning to read and write. April's phonological processing skills were within the average range. She was able to consistently rhyme and blend sounds together. She is beginning to understand how to delete sounds, identify sounds within words, and segment words into sounds. Her skills on this assessment match what Mrs. Patience has seen in the classroom.

There are two Diagnostic Clusters within the DAS-2, including Working Memory and Processing Speed. The Processing Speed cluster is a measure of general cognitive processing speed and reflects a student's ability to work with speed and accuracy. This cluster includes the Speed of Information Processing subtest, a measure of quickness in performing simple visual mental operations, and the Rapid Naming subtest, a measure of automaticity in integrating visual symbols with verbal naming. During both subtests, April worked accurately and at a steady pace. April's performance in this cluster was in the average range.

The Working Memory cluster is a measure of working memory, including short-term auditory and visual memory. Working Memory is a process underlying many cognitive abilities. It is the ability to use effective strategies to transform information or problem solve with information that is being held in short-term memory. For example, listening to a verbally presented series of numbers and then repeating them backwards or decoding an unfamiliar word and keeping each syllable in memory until you are ready to blend the sounds together. The Working Memory cluster includes the Recall of Digits Backwards and Recall of Sequential Order subtests. April used a good problem-solving strategy of repeating the information to help her remember. April's overall performance in the Working Memory cluster was in the average range.

Does April qualify for and need Special Education services to make progress toward grade-level academic standards?

April is currently receiving at-risk Resource Specialist Program (RSP) support. She is meeting many Kindergarten grade-level standards and does not currently demonstrate a learning disability. However, April meets Other Health Impairment (OHI) criteria. It is recommended that she be found eligible for Special Education services and continue her placement in a general education classroom with Resource Specialist Program (RSP) support.

April is a Kindergarten student enrolled in Current Unified School District at Smith Primary Academy. April was diagnosed with neurofibromatosis (NF1), a neurocutaneous genetic syndrome, at the age of 5 months. The severity of NF1 varies greatly and can present with different physical signs and complications for each person. April's mother has reported that her symptoms are currently mild and April's medical needs are monitored through a neurologist and orthopedist at Children's Hospital.

As many as 50% of students with NF1 demonstrate learning disabilities during their school years. Due to academic concerns of her parents and teacher, April was evaluated for possible learning disabilities. Based on the results of this evaluation, April is not currently demonstrating learning disabilities. Her cognitive processing abilities are all within the average range, though her verbal reasoning abilities are a relative strength. April initially made slow progress in mastering pre-reading and math skills during pre-Kindergarten and had difficulty retaining these over the summer. However, this school year she has received additional academic support through the Resource Specialist Program (RSP) and has made consistent and steady progress in learning and using beginning Kindergarten reading, written language, and math skills.

April has made strong academic progress and is meeting many Kindergarten standards. However, her NF1 symptoms and medical needs may change as she continues to develop, potentially affecting her academic achievement or educational performance. Therefore, it is recommended that April be found eligible for Special Education services under the eligibility criteria of *Other Health Impaired* (OHI). Students meet this eligibility if they have "limited strength, vitality or alertness, due to chronic or acute health problems which adversely affect a pupil's educational performance." April meets this eligibility because of her NF1 diagnosis and the continued medical monitoring she requires to stay healthy. An Individualized Education Program (IEP) meeting will convene to review these assessment results. Decisions regarding placement and services will be made by the IEP team.

Respectfully Submitted,
School Psychologist

Standardized Assessment Results

Two types of scores are presented below. Standard scores indicate where April's performance was on the assessment in relation to the mean or average score. April's performance is compared to students of the same age in the test's norming group. Standard scores from approximately 85 to 115 are within the average range. Scores lower than 85 are below average and higher than 115 are above average. Students' performance on tests can vary for many reasons; therefore, it may be inaccurate to describe a student's performance with a single standard score. The confidence interval is a band or range of scores, which is a more appropriate description of a student's performance. For these assessments a 95% confidence interval is presented, which can be interpreted as there being a 95% chance that April's true score falls within this range.

Differential Ability Scales (DAS-2) Early Years

Cluster	Subtest	Standard Score	Confidence Interval	Descriptive Category
Verbal		**113**	**103–120**	**Above Average**
	Naming Vocabulary			Above Average
	Verbal Comprehension			Above Average
Nonverbal Reasoning		**108**	**98–116**	**Average**
	Matrices			Average
	Picture Similarities			Above Average
Spatial		**84**	**80–90**	**Below Average**
	Pattern Construction			Average
	Copying			Low**
Working Memory		**93**	**87–100**	**Average**
	Recall of Sequential Order			Below Average
	Recall of Digits Backwards			Average
Processing Speed		**92**	**84–101**	**Average**
	Speed of Information Processing			**Average**
	Rapid Naming			**Average**

**These scores were unable to be appropriately interpreted. Please see the narrative regarding this assessment to better understand April's relative strengths and weaknesses.

**Example 5: Elementary Student, Initial Evaluation
Assessing for Autism**

*This is a referral-based, question-driven report in a domain-based report structure. It is
written at a 11.2 Flesch Kincaid grade level with 20% passive sentences.*

Student: Jacob Wells   **School:** Good Elementary
Gender: Male   **Primary Language:** English
Age: 6.3   **Current Placement:** Speech and Language
Grade: K

Reason for Referral: Since beginning Kindergarten this September, Jacob has
demonstrated expressive and receptive language delays, poor social skills, and
behavioral issues at school. Jacob was referred for further evaluation by the
Individualized Education Program (IEP) team during his initial Speech and Language
IEP meeting on November, DATE. During the SL evaluation, Jacob demonstrated
behaviors consistent with an autism spectrum disorder (ASD), including poor eye
contact, repetitive motor movements, and echolalia. The focus of this assessment is to
determine his eligibility and need for further special education services. Specifically,
this evaluation will answer the questions: What are Jacob's current cognitive processing
strengths and weaknesses? What are Jacob's academic skills relative to grade-level
language arts and math standards? How do Jacob's social skills, behavior, and
classroom adaptive skills impact his academic achievement? Do Jacob's current Special
Education eligibility and services meet his educational needs?

Assessment Procedures:

Review of Records:

Cumulative School Records	DATE
Classroom Work Samples	DATE
CUSD Behavioral Consultation Report	DATE

Interviews:

Jacob Wells, Student	DATE
Mrs. Wells, Mother	DATE
Mrs. Smith, Kindergarten Teacher	DATE

Observations:

Behavioral Assessment Scale for Children–3:	
Student Observation System (SOS)	DATE
Whole-Group Language Arts	DATE
Small-Group Math	DATE

Standardized Assessments:
Differential Ability Scales–2 (DAS-2)   DATE
Gilliam Autism Rating Scale: Teacher and Parent   DATE

Background Information: Jacob's background information was gathered through a review of his school records and interviews with both of his parents. Jacob is 6 years old and currently enrolled in Kindergarten at Good Elementary School. Jacob had limited school experience prior to enrolling in Kindergarten. According to Jacob's parents he attended three preschools for short periods of time. He was not academically, socially, or behaviorally successful in his preschool experiences. Mr. and Mrs. Wells expressed frustration that further resources and/or referrals for assistance were not provided prior to asking Jacob to leave the schools.

Jacob has attended school within Ideal Unified School District (CUSD) since enrolling in Kindergarten. He was initially assessed and found eligible for Speech and Language (SL) services in November of DATE. According to the SL report, Jacob exhibited the need for speech and language services due to a communication disorder in the area of semantics. Jacob has been receiving small-group SL services two times per week since his evaluation.

A health assessment was conducted as part of Jacob's initial Special Education evaluation. According to the school nurse's report, dated DATE, Jacob's vision was 20/30 when his right, left, and both eyes were tested. He passed the hearing screening and his immunizations are up to date. According to his mother, her pregnancy and birth with Jacob were normal. Jacob has received consistent medical care through his pediatrician. He did suffer a head injury and concussion at the age of 3. A CAT scan was completed, and no further treatment or concerns were noted. Overall, Jacob has been a healthy child.

According to Mrs. Wells, Jacob met developmental milestones within an age-appropriate range except for expressive and receptive language. According to his parents his first words occurred by 12 months of age, but Jacob did not put words together until 3½ years of age. They discussed their concerns with Jacob's pediatrician; however, the Wells' reported that the pediatrician was not concerned and told the family that "boys talk later than girls." Upon enrollment in Kindergarten, Jacob continued to demonstrate language difficulties at home and school. He often spoke in one- or two-word phrases, answered questions with off-topic information, or repeated phrases over and over.

Earlier this year Jacob's parents took him to Dr. Psych, a clinical psychologist, due to attention and behavior issues. Dr. Psych referred the family to Local Regional Center

(LRC) for further assessment in the areas of attention and suspected autism. Jacob's parents initiated an LRC referral, but were not satisfied with the agency's responses. Due to the academic and language progress he has made, as well as the services provided through the school, they have decided not to proceed with a service evaluation through LRC.

Evaluation Results:
Throughout the direct assessment, Jacob was cooperative and willing to participate. Jacob easily separated from his classroom when we conducted one-on-one assessments. Jacob was given time to look around the room and play with testing materials before we started. He was assessed during two 20–30-minute blocks of time over two days. Directions were repeated and extra practice items were used for all of the standardized assessment subtests. Jacob was redirected to task through verbal and physical prompts and a positive reinforcement system was used to earn time playing a game of choice after each testing session. With verbal and physical prompts to focus on the specific tasks and the use of the reinforcement system, he put forth good effort during all of the activities.

Cognitive Abilities:
Jacob's cognitive processing strengths and weaknesses were assessed through review of records, observations, teacher reports, interviews, and standardized measures. Based on these assessments, his overall cognitive ability is estimated to be within the broad average range.

According to his parents and classroom teacher, Jacob demonstrates an excellent memory for dramatic material. He has memorized lengthy dialogues from *Disney* films, as well as *Star Trek* episodes, and recites them with feeling. Although he often uses his recitation of the material inappropriately as a self-stimulating behavior or as an avoidance response to direct questions, his skills demonstrate a strong memory for information he hears. This school year Jacob has also demonstrated strong auditory memory skills through easily learning and remembering school songs.

During the assessment, Jacob appropriately engaged in imaginary play with a tea set, doll, and brush. When playing with the tea set, he used a British accent and formal language. For example, when asked if he would like more tea, he gave a serious nod and stated, "Of course, madam."

The Differential Abilities Scale (DAS-2) was also used to further evaluate Jacob's cognitive ability. The DAS-2 is a standardized nationally normed, individually administered assessment battery designed to evaluate cognitive processing in students 6 through 17 years, 11 months of age. Jacob was given selected subtests from the DAS-2 School Age Core Subtests. Cluster scores are estimates of overall functioning in broadly defined cognitive domains. Jacob's performance on the DAS varied greatly. The Verbal Cluster is composed of the Verbal Comprehension and Naming Vocabulary. Jacob's overall performance on this cluster was within the below-average range. Jacob was able to respond to single-step requests such as, "Show me Teddy's eyes" and "Put the horse in the box." He had more difficulty when simultaneous requests were given such as, "When I put down the tree, pick up the car." In the Naming Vocabulary subtest, Jacob was asked to identify pictures. Once he got to unfamiliar pictures he used his imagination to make up a word to go with the picture, such as "rincon" for *lock,* "muna" for *hourglass,* and "pifer" for *funnel.* Jacob's performance on the Verbal Cluster of the DAS is a reflection of his documented expressive language delays. Jacob worked best when minimal language processing was required. His performance on both the Pattern Construction subtest, from the Spatial cluster, and the Matrixes subtest, from the Non-Verbal cluster, were within the average range. The Matrixes subtest requires the student to select one out of four options that complete a puzzle, or matrix. On the Pattern Construction subtest, Jacob used multisided blocks to recreate single-dimension pictures. He enjoyed this activity though he worked slowly. The non-timed alternative scoring method was used when evaluating his performance. Jacob was very persistent with these subtests even when they became more difficult. His performance within these nonverbal areas is more indicative of his overall cognitive ability.

Academic Achievement:
Jacob's current academic achievement was assessed through review of records, observations, teacher reports, interviews, work samples, and curriculum-based assessments.

Pre-academic/Academic Skills: Jacob entered Kindergarten with many basic skills. On his initial Kindergarten skills screening he was able to identify 11/12 colors and 4/6 basic shapes. Jacob recognized numbers 1–15 and was able to rote count from 1 to 29. He identified 47/54 letter names, but knew no letter sounds. He also identified 2/36 sight-words and inconsistently wrote his first name.

Language Arts: Jacob has made academic progress this school year. On his latest literacy assessment Jacob correctly identified all letter names and 25/26 letter sounds. Jacob has been observed during Open Court reading. He has difficulty staying focused and on-task during whole-group instruction and independent work, though he will actively participate when the class sings and does the hand motions for the letter-sound cards. Jacob now identifies 32/36 Kindergarten sight-words and 15/25 high-frequency sight-words. The table shows Jacob's growth in these areas:

	Percent Correct	
	September of DATE	March of DATE
Letter names	87	100
Letter sounds	0	96
K sight-words	5	88

Jacob passed the pre-Kindergarten reading benchmark, a measure of basic book concepts and comprehension of a picture story, on DATE. He correctly demonstrated 5/5 concepts about print and answered 4/5 comprehension questions. Jacob was given the mid-Kindergarten reading benchmark on DATE, though he did not pass. His decoding accuracy was 87% and he answered 3/5 comprehension questions correctly. Jacob's decoding errors were contextual, as he used picture clues, not phonics, to read some of the words. For example, he read *bus* as "school bus" and *slide* as "playground." In phonemic awareness testing, Jacob has demonstrated rhyming, blending, and segmenting skills.

Jacob has demonstrated the ability to encode sounds when he receives one-on-one guidance. Initially, when given writing assignments, Jacob would draw a picture then scribble or write letter and number strands to accompany his picture. He still engages in this when writing in whole-group activities. With adult assistance Jacob will draw a picture and dictate 1–2 sentences. With one-on-one prompting, he is able to segment his words into sounds and write many of the words he dictates to the teacher.

Math: Jacob recently received a score of 80% (proficient) on his second trimester math assessment measuring counting to 20, size, and volume. He also scored an 80% (proficient) on his most recent addition assessment. Jacob is grasping addition and subtraction concepts and writing basic number sentences to match picture clues. Jacob's attention can negatively impact his one-to-one correspondence when counting. His best work is demonstrated in small groups where he can have redirection when needed.

Social and Behavioral Skills:
Jacob's social skills and behavior were assessed through interviews, observations, and standardized rating scales. Both Mrs. Smith, the classroom teacher, and Jacob's parents were asked to complete the Gilliam Autism Rating Scale (GARS). The GARS is a behavioral checklist created to help identify persons with autism spectrum disorders.

Behaviors are sorted into subtests, which correspond to specific characteristics of autism spectrum disorders: Stereotyped Behaviors, Communication, and Social Interaction. A standard score is given that represents the probability that a child has autism. Based on Jacob's parents' ratings, a standard score of 115 was given. This can be interpreted as his parents perceiving the probability of autism to be above average. Jacob's classroom teacher's ratings produced a standard score of 109, which can be interpreted as the probability of autism being high average to above average. Both Jacob's teacher's and parents' responses were significant in the areas of stereotyped behaviors and communication. They all believe that these are the areas where Jacob demonstrates the most unique behaviors.

Jacob demonstrates some stereotyped behaviors within the classroom and at home. Within the classroom Jacob will repeatedly spin in a circle or lay on the floor. At times he will rock back and forth when seated. Jacob often walks on his toes and moves erratically when going from place to place in the room. These behaviors have decreased over the year, though continue to occur at least once per day. Jacob continues to engage in vocalizations which often include repeating dialogue from his favorite shows or movies. His parents have noted a decrease in his vocalizations at home, though they still occur two to three times per hour.

Jacob rarely initiates or engages in conversation. He has recently begun to make a statement toward others, though he often leaves the interaction before he receives a response. Jacob will repeat words and phrases out of context and will respond to questions with off-topic statements. These behaviors have been observed with adults and peers in multiple school situations. Jacob's best conversational communication occurs in a quiet one-on-one setting where the speaker has his full attention. Language improvements have been noted by his teacher. Jacob has learned to greet and say good-bye to people and if focused will try to answer questions. During an observation, Jacob sneezed and the student sitting next to him said "Bless you." Jacob smiled and stated "Thank you." Jacob's mother has recently noted that at home he is providing more direct and on-topic answers when questioned about activities and events within his day.

Jacob typically does not initiate appropriate social interactions with peers. He has been observed initiating interaction through touching or off-topic statements within the classroom, and rough play at recess. Jacob does watch his peers and follows their actions as prompts for activity transitions in the classroom. Jacob appears to prefer not to make direct eye contact with adults, but will when engaged in a one-on-one conversation or when given a verbal or physical prompt. According to his parents, Jacob does not initiate interactions with peers in settings outside of the home, such as the park or in group swimming lessons. He prefers to play on his own. At home Jacob actively seeks out interactions with his family. He likes to play with his 12-year-old sister, will seek out a parent to read a book to him, and enjoys rougher games such as chase, tag, and wrestling. Jacob's father stated that they have recently moved into a larger home. Jacob enjoys playing outside and working with his dad in the garage.

Adaptive Skills:

Jacob's classroom adaptive behavior and home adaptive behavior were assessed through interviews and observations. In the classroom, Jacob's short attention span negatively impacts both his academic achievement and performance. He needs consistent prompts to stay focused and on-task. In a structured observation, Jacob demonstrated inattentive behaviors during 63% of the 15-minute observation. He responded to teacher prompts to return to his activity, but was often off-task again within 30 seconds. On a second observation, Jacob sat quietly with his legs crossed and hands folded in his lap throughout a 25-minute whole-group lesson, though he was rarely focused on the teacher. During the observation, Jacob stared at pictures on the walls.

At home, Jacob is appropriately independent in his self-care. He uses the restroom, bathes, feeds, and dresses himself. He will ask for assistance if he needs something, but prefers to try to get it on his own first. Jacob does demonstrate limited knowledge or understanding of danger in the community. He needs assistance crossing the street and supervision when outside. At school, Jacob independently uses the restroom and cafeteria. He needs assistance to get to and from his classroom, the office, and his speech room.

Summary:

Jacob is a 6-year-old student enrolled in Kindergarten at Good Elementary School. Jacob currently receives Speech and Language services due to expressive language delays. His current eligibility for services is Speech and Language Impairment. This assessment was completed to evaluate Jacob's current eligibility and need for further Special Education services.

The California Special Education Code states a student qualifies under the eligibility of Autistic-Like Behaviors if the pupil exhibits any combination of the following autistic-like behaviors that adversely affect educational performance, to include but not limited to: (1) an inability to use oral language for appropriate communication; (2) a history of extreme withdrawal or relating to people inappropriately, and continued impairment in social interaction from infancy through early childhood; (3) an obsession to maintain sameness; (4) extreme preoccupation with objects or inappropriate use of objects or both; (5) extreme resistance to controls; (6) displays peculiar motoric mannerisms and motility patterns; (7) self-stimulating, ritualistic behavior.

APPENDIX II

Based on the information gathered for this evaluation Jacob consistently exhibits five of the listed autistic-like behaviors at various degrees. Jacob has a history and continues to demonstrate delays in oral language. Jacob demonstrates impairments in social interactions with peers and adults that have been observed throughout his development. Jacob has demonstrated a strong preoccupation with specific movies and television shows. He uses repetitive dialogue from the movies in a self-stimulating manner. At times, Jacob demonstrates difficulty with physical boundaries with his own body and peers. The behaviors noted above have decreased at home and school since Jacob has enrolled in school. He has made marked improvement in his expressive language, his interactions with adults, and his ability to follow routines within the classroom. Improvements in language and social skills have also been observed at home. Although improvement has been observed, these behaviors continue to negatively impact his academic achievement. Jacob requires further Special Education services to make progress in the general education curriculum. An Individualized Education Program (IEP) meeting will convene to review these assessment results. Decisions regarding both eligibility and services will be decided by the IEP team.

Behavioral recommendations are provided through consultation with the CUSD Behavior Support Team.

- Give frequent and immediate verbal praise when desired behavior occurs.
- Give behavioral redirections in short, simple statements. Wait for Jacob to comply with the redirection before returning to the activity or moving on.
- Give behavioral redirections in the form of statements rather than questions (e.g., "Please sit on your bottom" rather than "Will you please sit on your bottom?").
- Allow time for Jacob to process and comply with a direction prior to giving a second.
- Be consistent in behavioral expectations across staff members and activities.
- Be specific when redirecting undesirable behaviors. State the behavior you want to see rather than the behavior you don't want to see (e.g., "Still hands" rather than "Stop banging your hands").
- Allow Jacob choices in non-preferred activities to increase motivation to complete those tasks.
- Consistently and frequently use a behavior contract that addresses one or two specific, observable, and measurable behaviors. The contract should be implemented in at least 15-minute increments or at every activity transition.

Respectfully Submitted,
School Psychologist

Example 6: Elementary Bilingual Student, Triennial Evaluation
Reassessing Special Education Eligibility, Placement, and Services

This report is at a 12.2 Flesch Kincaid grade level with 20% passive sentences.

Student: Rebecca Tapia   **School:** Chapman Elementary School
Gender: Female   **Primary Language:** English/Spanish
Age: 8.10   **Current Placement:** MM SDC
Grade: 3

Rebecca is a third-grade student enrolled in Current Unified School District at Elementary School. Rebecca has received Special Education services through placement in a mild-to-moderate Special Day Class (MM SDC) with related services since her initial Special Education evaluation. Rebecca currently receives services under the eligibility of Specific Learning Disability (SLD). Rebecca has academic goals in written language, math computation, and applied math. She has a history of steady academic growth and is currently mainstreamed into a general education classroom for 90 minutes of daily language arts instruction. A triennial, or three-year, review of Rebecca's Special Education eligibility, placement, and services is being conducted at this time. This evaluation will answer the following questions:

- How does Rebecca's educational history affect her current educational achievement?
- What are Rebecca's current academic skills in the areas of reading, written language, and math?
- Are Rebecca's Special Education eligibility, placement, and services meeting her educational needs?

Assessment Procedures: The following procedures were chosen to provide data and information to assist in answering the evaluation questions. Based on a review of records and interviews with her grandmother and teachers, further standardized assessment was not needed to answer the evaluation questions.

Review of Records:

Cumulative School Records	DATE
Classroom Work Samples	DATE
CUSD Criterion-Based Assessments	DATE

APPENDIX II

Interviews:
    Special Education Teacher, Selena Class   DATE
    General Education Teacher, Zoe Right   DATE
    Guardian, Constance Tapia   DATE
    Speech and Language Therapist, Julia Word   DATE
Observations:
    Recess   DATE
    Small-Group Math Instruction   DATE

Assessment Questions and Results: After each question, the answer is provided in bold and italics. The information and data used to answer the question are also provided.

How does Rebecca's educational history impact her current educational achievement?

Rebecca was born prematurely and had significant early medical needs. She received early intervention services through Local Regional Center (LRC) from birth to 3 years of age. She has received Special Education services since her initial evaluation at the age of 3. Rebecca has made steady and consistent academic growth, meeting 80% of her overall annual IEP goals.

Rebecca's background information was gathered through a review of her cumulative records and an interview with her grandmother, Constance Tapia. Rebecca was born at 25 weeks' gestation. She had significant medical needs and was in the neonatal intensive care unit for 4½ months.

Rebecca received early intervention services through Local Regional Center (LRC) when she was released from the hospital. These services included in-home infant stimulation, physical therapy, and speech and language therapy. Rebecca's first language was English, though Spanish was spoken in the home between caregivers. Rebecca's early therapies were all conducted in English, though her mother noted that her grandmother, who lived with them, only spoke Spanish to Rebecca.

Rebecca was referred to Current Unified School District (CUSD) for an evaluation for Special Education eligibility and services before her third birthday. Rebecca was evaluated in English and Spanish, though English was identified as her dominant language. According to the initial evaluation she demonstrated strengths in cognitive and social development and delays in language, visual, and fine-motor development. She was found eligible for services under the Developmental Delay (DD) criteria.

164

An Individualized Education Plan (IEP) was held on DATE and educational goals were created in the areas of attention, number relationships, writing, and expressive language. Rebecca began attending preschool at Chapman Elementary School in their Special Day Class (SDC) for students with mild-to-moderate (MM) disabilities. She also began receiving 60 weekly minutes each of Speech and Language (SL) and Occupational Therapy (OT) services.

Annual IEP meetings were held in December of DATE and DATE. Rebecca made academic progress, meeting 75% of her IEP goals. Her services, including placement in the SDC preschool, SL, and OT, remained the same. She transitioned into Chapman's Kindergarten/first-grade MM SDC for Kindergarten and began mainstreaming into a general education Kindergarten classroom for 60 minutes of daily language arts instruction.

A triennial assessment of Rebecca's Special Education eligibility, placement, and services was held in November of Kindergarten. According to the psychoeducational evaluation report, Rebecca's overall cognitive ability was in the average range. She had weaknesses in nonverbal reasoning and strengths in verbal reasoning. According to the Occupational Therapy (OT) assessment, Rebecca continued to have difficulty with visual motor tracking, coordinating distal movements, and bilateral coordination, which negatively impacted her fine-motor skills and visual motor coordination. The Speech and Language (SL) therapist reported that Rebecca had age-appropriate voice quality, fluency, and articulation. Her expressive and receptive language was in the average and she had met all of her SL goals.

Based on results from the psychoeducational, OT, and SL evaluations, the IEP team decided to change Rebecca's Special Education eligibility to Specific Learning Disability (SLD). Her cognitive abilities were estimated to be in the average range. She demonstrated relative weaknesses in visual motor integration and motor planning. These weaknesses were impacting her academic achievement in written language, math computation, and applied math. Her placement remained the MM SDC with mainstreaming for language arts instruction. She also received 60 minutes of weekly OT services and 30 minutes of monthly SL consultation.

Rebecca continued mainstreaming into a general education Kindergarten classroom, though the time was increased to 90 minutes a day. She continued to makes solid progress and completed Kindergarten, passing the Middle of Kindergarten literacy screenings, measures of letter-sound knowledge and sight-words. She also passed the End of Kindergarten fiction reading benchmark, a measure of reading fluency and comprehension.

Rebecca continued in the Kindergarten/first-grade MM SDC for first grade with 60 weekly minutes of OT and 90 minutes of daily mainstreaming. At her annual IEP, Rebecca had met 80% of her goals. Rebecca completed first grade, passing the End of First Grade fiction and nonfiction reading benchmarks and the End of Kindergarten phonemic awareness literacy screening. With extended time as an accommodation, she was proficient in addition and subtraction facts to 10.

Rebecca transitioned into the second-/third-grade MM SDC for second grade. At her annual IEP meeting Rebecca again met 80% of her goals. Her services in OT and mainstreaming remained the same. Rebecca took the State Standards Tests (SST) for the first time as a second-grader. Rebecca scored in the *Far Below Basic* range in Math and the *Basic* range in ELA. She continued in the second-/third-grade MM SDC for third grade where she is currently receiving 60 minutes a week of OT and is mainstreamed for language arts instruction every day for 90 minutes.

Rebecca's primary language continues to be English and her instruction and related service therapies have always been provided in English. Rebecca's primary caregiver is currently her grandmother, whose primary language is Spanish. Rebecca speaks both English and Spanish at home with her grandmother. Her grandmother was interviewed in Spanish and noted that Rebecca's expressive Spanish skills have improved. They are both teaching each other their primary languages and she is impressed at how well Rebecca Spanish is improving.

What are Rebecca's current academic skills in the areas of reading, written language, and math?

Rebecca's current academic achievement was assessed through review of records, observations, teacher reports, interviews, observations, classroom work samples, and criterion-based assessments. Rebecca is a responsible, motivated, and hardworking student who is a pleasure to have in class. Overall, Rebecca is meeting many grade-level standards in reading. Her writing format and content has also progressed. Math computation is an academic challenge for Rebecca.

Language Arts: CUSD uses reading benchmarks to assess students' reading mastery. Reading benchmarks are given when the teacher believes the student has demonstrated the literacy skills to pass the reading assessment at a specific level. Rebecca passed the End of Second Grade nonfiction benchmark last June. Mrs. Class, her Special Education teacher, and Ms. Right, her mainstreaming teacher, noted that Rebecca has strong phonemic awareness and decoding skills. She is able to comprehend what she reads. Her ability to answer literal and inferential comprehension questions and summarize text is at grade level. These skills continue to be an academic strength for Rebecca.

On a recent unedited writing activity about Halloween, Rebecca wrote: "Halloween is really scary. Firct Bats are sscary and Furry. Next I go trick or treating. I get Candy Apples. They feel like marshmelows. Last There are PumPkins. I like Halloween."

Rebecca has good ideas for her writing and is able to organize her ideas using a prewriting tool such as mapping. She is able to form her ideas into basic sentences and a paragraph using an introductory sentence, transition words, and an ending sentence. Her penmanship has improved, though she continues to work on proper spacing and mixes upper- and lowercase letters in her writing. She uses her strong phonics skills to spell unknown words.

Math: Math is a more challenging subject for Rebecca. Rebecca has had difficulty memorizing basic math facts. Rebecca uses a number line to help her count up or backwards when completing math computations. When given an accommodation of extended time, Rebecca is partially proficient on CUSD addition math facts tests to 20. She is working on her proficiency in subtraction. Rebecca is more confident and successful with applied math. When given a single-step word problem, she is able to identify the operation to use and create a number sentence. Rebecca is currently being introduced to multiplication. She learns best when math concepts are previewed and reviewed in small groups. She needs repeated teaching and review to master new math concepts.

Classroom Adaptive Skills: According to Mrs. Class and Ms. Right, Rebecca is a responsible and hardworking student. She participates in classroom discussions and contributes to class lessons. Rebecca is able to start tasks in a timely manner, though she sometimes needs extra time to complete her work. She consistently completes all of her classwork and returns all of her homework. Rebecca is an overall motivated student who wants to learn and enjoys her time at school. Rebecca is very social with peers and is respectful to adults. She has many friends and is able to successfully interact with her classmates in many different classroom and recess situations. She is an overall happy child who enjoys school and interacting with others.

Are Rebecca's current Special Education eligibility, placement, and services meeting her educational needs?

Rebecca has received Special Education services under the Specific Learning Disability (SLD) eligibility since her triennial IEP in December of DATE. Rebecca continues to make good-to-steady progress in all academic areas. Based on the results of this evaluation, her current eligibility, placement, and services are meeting her educational needs, though it is recommended that the IEP team consider increasing Rebecca's mainstreaming time during social studies, science, and non-core academic activities.

Rebecca's current academic achievement was assessed through review of records, observations, teacher reports, interviews, classroom work samples, and criterion-based assessments. Rebecca is a responsible, motivated, and hardworking student who is a pleasure to have in class. Overall, Rebecca is meeting many grade-level standards in reading. Her writing format and content has also progressed. Math is an academic challenge for Rebecca. Rebecca has continued to make good-to-steady progress in all academic areas. Based on the current OT assessment, delays in visual motor integration and motor planning continue to impact Rebecca's academic achievement.

Rebecca's teachers have reported that Rebecca is a responsible, motivated, and hardworking student. She is socially successful with peers and adults in a variety of school settings. Based on the results of this evaluation, Rebecca's current eligibility, placement, and services are meeting her educational needs. Rebecca's IEP team, including her teachers and grandmother, hope to transition Rebecca to general education with Special Education math support by the time she is in fifth grade. The SDC environment provides Rebecca with the specialized instruction and extra time she needs to make progress toward grade-level standards. However, based on her grade-level literacy skills and developing writing skills it is recommended that Rebecca's mainstreaming be increased to include social studies and science, as well as all non-core academic activities. This will help support her transition to general education, while allowing her specialized support during math and small-group writing instruction. An Individualized Education Program (IEP) meeting will convene to review these evaluation results. Decisions regarding eligibility, placement, and services will be made by the IEP team.

Respectfully Submitted,
School Psychologist

Interview Protocol

The following questions are structured as if you were asking the student these questions. Feel free to change the wording so that it would fit an interview with a parent or teacher.

Home/Family:

1. Whom do you live with? (If there is a non-custodial parent, find out what the visitation schedule is.)
2. Family living outside the home?

Health:

3. Recent doctor visits?
4. Significant illnesses or injuries?
5. Medication? Now or in the past?
6. Vision and hearing?

Motor Skills:

7. Handwriting and fine-motor skills?
8. Participation in sports and gross motor skills?

Education/School:

9. Current school? Grade or level?
10. School history, including preschool?
11. Favorite classes or subjects?

12. Most difficult classes or subjects?
13. Do you get any extra help with these subjects? Who helps you? How do they help you?
14. Recent grades?
15. Experiences with homework? (How does the student experience homework? Is it difficult, easy, etc.? About how much homework does the student complete in a day or week? Try to get a percentage.)

Activities and Self: Interests, Skills, and Engagement in Productive Activities:

16. What are some things you like to do or think that you are good at?
17. How do you like to spend your free time? What are ways you have of relaxing and having fun? Hobbies, sports, music/movies?
18. How do you relax and have fun with your family (including common interests and activities)?

Coping:

19. How do you calm yourself down when upset or angry?
20. How do you handle difficult or stressful situations? Give an example of the last difficult situation you faced and how you handled it.

Social Support and Role Models:

21. What are your friends like (ages, gender)? What are some things you like to do together?
22. Whom are you closest to in your family?
23. When you get into trouble at home, how do your parents handle it?
24. Who in your life helps you reach your goals or explore your interests?
25. Name some people whom you respect or whom you see doing things you like or appreciate. What kinds of things do they do?

Required Helpfulness:

26. Who counts on you? (Follow up with: What do you do for them?)
27. Tell me about a time you did something nice for someone else, or you helped someone, or you gave him or her something they needed. What types of things do you enjoy doing for others?
28. How do you help out around the house?

Participation in Community:

29. Do you belong to any clubs, teams, community organizations, or churches (synagogues, temples, etc.)?

Goals and Aspirations:

30. If things went well for you over the next month, what would be different?
31. How do you see yourself in a year?
32. How about when you are an adult?

Transitions:

33. Did you recently change schools or are you planning to change schools?
34. Have you changed houses or are you planning to move soon?
35. Have there been any big changes in your family recently?

"Waking Day" Interview:

36. Think of a regular day for you. Tell me what you do first thing when you get up. What's next? And after that? (Have the child describe what he or she does from waking up to going to bed at night.)

Screening for Social-Emotional Problems:

37. Have you been feeling sad or angry lately? (Depression)
38. Have you lost interest in or stopped enjoying the things that you usually like to do? (Depression)
39. Have you ever thought your life was not worth living or thought about hurting yourself in some way? (Depression)
40. How is your appetite? What kinds of things do you like to eat? Have you gained or lost weight lately? (Depression)
41. How do you sleep? About how much do you sleep each night? (Depression)
42. Do you often have trouble paying attention to details or keeping your mind on what you are doing? (ADHD)
43. Are you told to sit still a lot? (ADHD)
44. Do you usually get upset and lose your temper if things don't go your way? (ODD)
45. Do you talk back or argue with your parents a lot? Your teachers? (ODD)
46. Do you worry more than other kids your age? If so, do you worry as often as every day or every other day? What do you worry about? (Anxiety)

Summary Sheet/Global Impressions:

47. Significant strengths or areas of typical functioning
48. Areas of significant need and risks
49. Suspected disabilities
50. Actions needed to enhance strengths and reduce risk

References

American Educational Research Association, American Psychological Association, & National Council on Measurement in Education. (2013). *Standards for educational and psychological testing*. Washington, DC: American Educational Research Association.

American Psychological Association. (2006). *Publication manual of the American Psychological Association* (6th ed.). Washington, DC: Author.

Andrews, L. W., & Gutkin, T. B. (1994). Influencing attitudes regarding special class placement using a psychoeducational report: An investigation of the elaboration likelihood model. *Journal of School Psychology, 32*, 321–337.

Assistance to States for Education of Children with Disabilities Program and the Preschool Grants for Children with Disabilities Program. (2006). CFR Sec. 300.8(c)(1)(i).

Bagnato S. J. (1980). The efficacy of diagnostic reports as individualized guides to prescriptive goal planning. *Exceptional Children, 46*, 554–557.

Batsche, G. (1983). The referral oriented, consultative assessment report writing model. In *Communicating psychological information in writing*. Retrieved from ERIC database (ED 240775).

Benard, B. (2004). *Resiliency: What we have learned*. San Francisco, CA: WestEd.

Bradley-Johnson, S., & Johnson, C. M. (2006). *A handbook for writing effective psychoeducational reports* (2nd ed.). Austin, TX: Pro-Ed.

Brandt, H. M., & Giebink, J. W. (1968). Concreteness and congruence in psychologists' reports to teachers. *Psychology in the Schools, 5*, 87–89.

Brenner, E. (2003), Consumer-focused psychological assessment. *Professional Psychology: Research and Practice, 34*, 240–247.

Brown-Chidsey, R., & Steege, M. W. (2005). Solution-focused psychoeducational reports. In R. Brown-Chidsey (Ed.), *Assessment for intervention: A problem solving approach* (pp. 267–290). New York, NY: Guilford Press.

California Education Code. (2009). Section 56320–56331. Retrieved from http://law.justia .com/california/codes/edc/56320–56331.html.

Carriere, J. A., Kennedy, K. K., & Hass, M. (2013). *Effectiveness of Psychoeducational Report Models*. Manuscript submitted for publication.

Cason, E. B. (1945). Some suggestions on the interaction between the school psychologist and the classroom teacher. *Journal of Counseling Psychology, 9*, 132–137.

Cook, W. A. (1912). A brief survey of the development of compulsory education in the United States. *The Elementary School Teacher, 12*(7), 331–335.

Cornwall, A. (1990). Social validation of psychoeducational assessment reports. *Journal of Learning Disabilities, 23*, 413–416.

Curtis, M. J., Hunley, S. A., & Grier, J. E. (2002). Relationships among the professional practices and demographic characteristics of school psychologists. *School Psychology Review, 31*(1), 30–43.

Davidson, I. F. W. K., & Simmons, J. N. (1991). Assessment reports: A preliminary study of teachers' perceptions. *B.C. Journal of Special Education, 15*, 247–253.

Donders, J. (1999). Pediatric neuropsychological reports: Do they really have to be so long? *Child Neuropsychology, 5*, 70–78.

Donovan, S. A., & Nickerson, A. B. (2007). Strength-based versus traditional social-emotional reports: Impact on multidisciplinary team members' perceptions. *Behavioral Disorders, 32*(4), 228–237.

Eberst, N. D., & Genshaft, J. (1984). Differences in school psychological report writing as a function of doctoral vs. nondoctoral training. *Psychology in the Schools, 21*(1), 78–82.

Epstein, M. H., Harniss, M. K., Robbins, V., Wheeler, L., Cyrulik, S., Kriz, M., & Nelson, R. (2003). Strength-based approaches to assessment in schools. In M. D. Weist, S. W. Evans, & N. A. Lever (Eds.), *Handbook of school mental health: Advancing practice and research* (pp. 285–300). New York, NY: Kluwer Academic/Plenum.

Epstein, M. H., Hertzog, M. A., & Reid, R. (2001). The behavioral and emotional rating scale: Long term test–retest reliability. *Behavioral Disorders, 26*(4), 314–320.

Fagan, T. K. (1990). A brief history of school psychology in the United States. In A. Thomas & J. Grimes (Eds.), *Best practices in school psychology* (pp. 913–929). Washington, DC: National Association of School Psychologists.

Fagan, T. K., & Wise, P. S. (2000). *School psychology: Past, present, and future*. Bethesda, MD: National Association of School Psychologists.

Farling, W. H. (1976, 09). *School psychology 1976: Old problems and new opportunities*. Paper presentation at the meeting of the Annual Conference of the American Psychological Association, Washington, DC.

References

Farling, W. H., & Hoedt, K. C. (1971). *National, regional, and state survey of school psychologists*. Retrieved from ERIC database (ED 061553).

Federal Register/Vol. 71, No. 156/Monday, August 14, 2006/Rules and Regulations, p. 4661.

Figueroa, R. A., & Newsome, P. (2006). The diagnosis of LD in English learners: Is it nondiscriminatory? *Journal of Learning Disabilities, 39*, 206–214.

Flanagan, D. P., & Harrison, P. L. (2005). *Contemporary intellectual assessment: Theories, tests and issues* (2nd ed.). New York, NY: Guilford Press.

Flesch, R. (1948). A new readability yardstick. *Journal of Applied Psychology, 32*, 231–233.

Frey, N. (2005). Retention, social promotion, and academic red-shirting: What do we know and need to know? *Remedial and Special Education, 26*(6), 332–346.

Gilman, R., & Medway, F. J. (2007). Teachers' perceptions of school psychology: A comparison of regular and special education teacher ratings. *School Psychology Quarterly, 22*(2), 145–161.

Goldwasser, E., Meyers, J., Christenson, S., & Graden, J. (1983). The impact of PL 94-142 on the practice of school psychology: A national survey. *Psychology in the Schools, 20*, 153–165.

Hagborg, W. J., & Aiello-Coultier, M. (1994). Teacher's perceptions of psychologists' reports of assessment. *Perceptual and Motor Skills, 78*, 171–176.

Harvey, V. S. (1997). Improving readability of psychological reports. *Professional Psychology, Research and Practice, 28*, 271–274.

Harvey, V. S. (2006). Variables affecting the clarity of psychological reports. *Journal of Clinical Psychology, 62*(1), 5–18.

Hutton, J. B., Dubes, R., & Muir, S. (1992). Assessment practices of school psychologists: Ten years later. *School Psychology Review, 21*, 271–284.

Individuals with Disabilities Education Act (IDEA). (2004). Sec. 300.306, *Determination of eligibility*. Retrieved from http://idea.ed.gov/explore/view/p/,root,regs,300,D,300%252E306.

Individuals with Disabilities Education Act (IDEA). (2004). Sec. 300.304, *Evaluation procedures*. Retrieved from http://idea.ed.gov/explore/view/p/%2Croot%2Cregs%2C300%2CD%2C300%252E304%2C

Kamphaus, R. W., DiStefano, C., Dowdy, E., Eklund, K., & Dunn, A. R. (2010). Determining the presence of a problem: Comparing two approaches for detecting youth behavioral risk. *School Psychology Review, 39*, 395–407.

King, S. (2000). *On writing: A memoir of the craft*. New York: Simon & Schuster.

Klare, G. R. (1976). A second look at the validity of readability formulas. *Journal of Reading Behavior, 8*(2), 129–52.

Klare, G. R., Mabry, J. E., & Gustafson, L. M. (1955). The relationship of style difficulty to immediate retention and to acceptability of technical material. *Journal of Educational Psychology, 46*, 287–295.

Klare, G. R., Shuford, E. H., & Nichols, W. H. (1957). The relationship of style difficulty, practice, and efficiency of reading and retention. *Journal of Applied Psychology, 41,* 222–226.

Klopfer, W. G. (1960). *The psychological report: Use and communication of psychological findings.* New York, NY: Grune & Stratton.

Kutner, M., Greenberg, E., Jin, Y., Boyle, B., Hsu, Y., & Dunleavy, E. (2007). *Literacy in everyday life: Results from the 2003 National Assessment of Adult Literacy.* Washington, DC: National Center for Education Statistics, Institute of Education Sciences, U.S. Department of Education.

Lau, M. Y., & Blatchey, L. A. (2009). A comprehensive, multidimensional approach to assessment of culturally and linguistically diverse students. In J. M. Jones (Ed.), *The psychology of multiculturalism in the schools: A primer for practice, training, and research* (pp. 139–171). Bethesda, MD: NASP.

Leung, B. (1993). Back to basics: Assessment is a R.I.O.T.! *NASP Communiqué, 22*(3), 1–6. Retrieved from http://www.nasponline.org/publications/cq/.

Levitt, V. H., & Merrell, K. W. (2009). Linking assessment to intervention for internalizing problems of children and adolescents. *School Psychology Forum, 3*(1), 13–26.

Lichtenberger, E. O., Mather, N., Kaufman, N. L., & Kaufman, A. S. (2004). *Essentials of assessment report writing.* Hoboken, NJ: John Wiley & Sons.

Lidz, C. (2006). The therapeutic misconception and our models of competency and informed consent. *Behavioral Sciences & the Law, 24,* 535–546.

Lopez, S. J., Snyder, C. R., & Rasmussen, H. N. (2003). Striking a vital balance: Developing a complementary focus on human weakness and strength through positive psychological treatment. In S. J. Lopez & C. R. Snyder (Eds.), *Positive psychological assessment: A handbook of models and measures* (pp. 3–20). Washington, DC: American Psychological Association.

Lostutter, M. (1947). Some critical factors in newspaper readability. *Journalism Quarterly, 24,* 307–314.

Mastoras, S. M., Climie, E. A., McCrimmon, A. W., & Schwean, V. L. (2011, June). A C.L.E.A.R. approach to report writing: A framework for improving the efficacy of psychoeducational reports. *Canadian Journal of School Psychology, 26,* 127–147. doi:10.1177/0829573511409722

McBride, G., Dumont, R., & Willis, J. O. (2011). *Essentials of IDEA for assessment professionals.* New York, NY: John Wiley & Sons.

Merrell, K. W., Ervin, R. A., & Gimpel, G. A. (2006). *School psychology for the 21st century.* New York, NY: Guilford Press.

Michaels, M. H. (2006). Ethical considerations in writing psychological assessment reports. *Journal of Clinical Psychology, 62*(1), 47–58.

References

Minneapolis Public Schools. (2001). *Report of the external review committee on the Minneapolis Problem Solving Model.*

Murphy, D. (1947). How plain talk increases readership 45% to 60%. *Printer's Ink, 220,* 35–37.

Mussman, M. C. (1964). Teachers' evaluations of psychological reports. *Journal of School Psychology, 3,* 35–37.

National Association of School Psychologists. (1997). *Principles for professional ethics.* Bethesda, MD: Author.

National Association of School Psychologists. (2006). *School Psychology: A blueprint for training and practice III.* Retrieved from http://www.nasponline.org/resources/blueprint/FinalBlueprintInteriors.pdf.

National Association of School Psychologists. (2009). *NASP publications: Best practices in school psychology V.* Retrieved from http://www.nasponline.org/publications/booksproducts/BP5.aspx.

National Association of School Psychologists. (2010). *Professional conduct manual: Principles for professional ethics and guidelines for the provision of school psychological services.* Bethesda, MD: Author.

National Association of School Psychologists. (2010). Principles for Professional Ethics and Guidelines for the Provision of School Psychological Services. Retrieved from National Association of School Psychologists' website: http://www.nasponline.org/standards/2010standards.aspx

National Association of School Psychologists (n.d.). *What do school psychologists do?* Retrieved July 8, 2013, from http://www.nasponline.org/about_sp/whatis.aspx.

National Center on Response to Intervention. (2010). *Essential components of RTI: A closer look at response to intervention.* Washington, DC: U.S. Department of Education, Office of Special Education Programs, National Center on Response to Intervention. Retrieved from http://www.rti4success.org/images/stories/pdfs/rtiessentialcomponents_051310.pdf.

National Conference of State Legislators. (2007). *State and federal issues.* Retrieved from http://www.ncsl.org/programs/educ/CompulsoryEd.htm.

National Dissemination Center for Children with Disabilities. (2010). *Supports, modifications, and accommodations for students.* Retrieved August 16, 2013, from http://nichcy.org/schoolage/accommodations.

Nickerson, A. B. (2007). The use and importance of strength-based assessment. *School Psychology Forum: Research in Practice, 2,* 15–25. Retrieved from http://www.nasponline.org/publications/spf/issue2_1/nickerson.pdf.

Olvera, P., & Gomez-Cerrillo, L. (2011). A bilingual approach (English & Spanish) psycho-educational assessment model grounded in Cattell-Horn-Carroll (CHC) theory: A cross battery approach. *Contemporary School Psychology, 15,* 113–123.

Ortiz, S. O. (2008). Best practices in nondiscriminatory assessment. In A. Thomas & J. Grimes (Eds.), *Best practices in school psychology* (pp. 661–678). Bethesda, MD: National Association of School Psychologists.

Ortiz, S. O., Flanagan, D. P., & Dynda, A. M. (2008). Best practices in working with culturally diverse children and families. In A. Thomas & J. Grimes (Eds.), *Best practices in school psychology* (pp. 1721–1738). Bethesda, MD: National Association of School Psychologists.

Orwell, George (1950). *Shooting an elephant and other essays*. New York: Harcourt, Brace.

Ownby, R. L. (1997). *Psychological reports: A guide to report writing in professional psychology*. New York, NY: John Wiley & Sons.

Rafoth, M. A., & Richmond, B. O. (1983). Useful terms in psychoeducational reports: A survey of students, teachers, and psychologists. *Psychology in the Schools, 20*, 346–350.

Raines, T., Dever, B., Kamphaus, R., & Roach, A. (2012). Universal screening for behavioral and emotional risk: A promising method for reducing disproportionate placement in special education. *Journal of Negro Education, 81*(3), 283–296.

Reschley, D. J. (2000). The present and future status of school psychology in the United States. *School Psychology Review, 29*, 507–522.

Rhodes, R. L., Ochoa, S. H., & Ortiz, S. O. (2005). *Assessing culturally and linguistically diverse students: A practical guide*. New York, NY: Guilford Press.

Ross-Reynolds, G. (1990). Best practices in report writing. In A. Thomas & J. Grimes (Eds.), *Best practices in school psychology II* (pp. 621–633). Bethesda, MD: National Association of School Psychologists.

Salvagno, M., & Teglasi, H. (1987). Teacher perceptions of different types of information in psychological reports. *Journal of School Psychology, 25*, 415–424.

Salvia, J. A., & Ysseldyke, J. E. (2001). *Assessment in special and remedial education* (8th ed.). Boston, MA: Houghton Mifflin.

Salvia, J., Ysseldyke, J. E., & Bolt, S. (2007). *Assessment in special and inclusive education* (10th ed.). Boston, MA: Houghton Mifflin.

Sattler, J. M. (1992). *Assessment of children* (3rd ed.). San Diego, CA: Author.

Sattler, J. M. (2001). *Assessment of children: Cognitive applications* (4th ed.). La Mesa, CA: Author.

Sattler, J. M. (2008). *Assessment of children: Cognitive foundations* (5th ed.). La Mesa, CA: Author.

Schramm, W. (1947). Measuring another dimension of newspaper readership. *Journalism Quarterly, 24*, 293–306.

Seligman, M. E. P., & Csikszentmihalyi, M. (2000). Positive psychology: An introduction. *American Psychologist, 55*, 5–14.

Severson, H. H., Walker, H. M., Hope-Doolittle, J., Kratochwill, T. R., & Gresham, F. M. (2007). Proactive, early screening to detect behaviorally at-risk students: Issues, approaches, emerging innovations, and professional practices, *Journal of School Psychology*, *45*, 2, 193–223.

Shanteau, J., Weiss, Thomas & Pounds, (2003). How can you tell if someone is an expert?: Empirical assessment of expertise. In L. Sandra, S. L. Schneider, & J. Shanteau (Eds.), *Emerging perspectives on decision research* (pp.). Cambridge, UK: Cambridge University Press.

Shinn, M. R. (2002). Best practices in using curriculum-based measurement in a problem-solving model. In A. Thomas & J. Grimes (Eds.), *Best practices in school psychology IV* (pp. 671–697). Bethesda, MD: National Association of School Psychologists.

Smith, D. K. (1984). Practicing school psychologists: Their characteristics, activities and populations served. *Professional Psychology: Research and Practice, 15*, 798–810.

Snyder, C.R., & Elliott, T.R. (2005). Clinical psychology education in the 21st century: The four level matrix model. *Journal of Clinical Psychology, 61*, 1033–1054.

Snyder, C. R., Ritschel, L., Rand, K. L., & Berg, C. J. (2006). Balancing psychological assessments: Including strengths and hope in client reports. *Journal of Clinical Psychology, 62* (1), 33–46.

Sternberg, R. J. (1985). *Beyond IQ: A triarchic theory of intelligence*. Cambridge, UK: Cambridge University Press.

Swanson, C. E. (1948). Readability and readership: A controlled experiment. *Journalism Quarterly, 25*, 339–343.

Tallent, N. (1993). *Psychological report writing* (4th ed.). Englewood Cliffs, NJ: Prentice Hall.

Tallent, N., & Reiss, W. J. (1959). Multidisciplinary views on the preparation of written clinical psychological reports: The trouble with psychological reports. *Journal of Clinical Psychology, 15*, 444–446.

Tassé, M. J., Schalock, R. L., Balboni, G., Bersani, H. R., Borthwick-Duffy, S. A., Spreat, S., . . . Zhang, D. (2012). The construct of adaptive behavior: Its conceptualization, measurement, and use in the field of intellectual disability. *American Journal on Intellectual and Developmental Disabilities, 117*(4), 291–303. doi:10.1352/1944-7558-117.4.291

Teglasi, H. (1983). Report of a psychological assessment in a school setting. *Psychology in the Schools, 20*, 466–479.

Thomas, A., & Grimes, J. (Eds.). (1985). *Best practices in school psychology*. Washington, DC: National Association of School Psychologists.

Thomas, A., & Grimes, J. (Eds.). (2008). *Best practices in school psychology V*. Washington, DC: National Association of School Psychologists.

Tidwell, R., & Wetter, J. (1978). Parental evaluations of psychoeducational reports: A case study. *Psychology in the Schools, 15*(2), 209–215.

United States Department of Education. (2003). *National Assessment of Adult Literacy. Institute of Education Services. National Center for Education Statistics*. Retrieved from http://nces.ed.gov/naa

Weddig, R. A. (1984). Parental interpretation of psychoeducational reports. *Psychology in the Schools, 21*, 477–481.

Wiener, J. (1985). Teachers' comprehension of psychological reports. *Psychology in the Schools, 22*(1), 60–64.

Wiener, J. (1987). Factors affecting educators' comprehension of psychological reports. *Psychology in the Schools, 24*(2), 116–126.

Wiener, J., & Costaris, L. (2012). Teaching psychological report writing: Content and process. *Canadian Journal of School Psychology, 27*(2), 119–135.

Wiener, J., & Kohler, S. (1986). Parents' comprehension of psychological reports. *Psychology in the Schools, 23*, 265–270.

Wolber, G. J., & Carne, W. F. (2002). *Writing psychological reports: A guide for clinicians* (2nd ed.). Sarasota, FL: Professional Resource Press.

Wright, B. A., & Fletcher, B. L. (1982). Uncovering hidden resources: A challenge in assessment. *Professional Psychology, 13*, 229–235.

Yell, M. L. (1998). *The law and special education*. Columbus, OH: Merrill.

Ysseldyke, J., & Christenson, S. L. (2002). *Functional assessment of academic behavior*. Longmont, CO: Sopris West.

Author Index

Subject Index